D0191706

Scientific Advisory Board:

R. James Barnard, Ph.D., University of Iowa
Professor, University of California at Los Angeles, with appointments in the Department of Kinesiology and the School of Medicine. Former Vice President, American College of Sports Medicine, and United States Public Health Service Research Career Development Award recipient.

Diane Hanson, Ph.D., New York University, R.N.
Vice President of Pritikin Systems, Inc. Behavioral Specialist/ Educator, Pritikin Longevity Center. Contributing editor, *Journal of Health Promotion.*

Stephen B. Inkeles, M.D., Loyola University
Staff Physician, Pritikin Longevity Center. Clinical Instructor, University of California at Los Angeles School of Medicine, Division of Clinical Nutrition. Diplomate of the American Boards of Internal Medicine and Nutrition. Fellow of the American College of Nutrition.

James J. Kenney, Ph.D., Rutgers University, R.D.
Nutrition Research Specialist/Educator, Pritikin Longevity Center. Instructor, University of California at Los Angeles Department of Kinesiology. Diplomate of the American Board of Nutrition. Board of Directors of the National Council Against Health Fraud, and contributing editor, *Nutrition Forum.*

Monroe B. Rosenthal, M.D., Chicago Medical School
Medical Director of Pritikin Longevity Center. Diplomate of the American Board of Internal Medicine.

Denise Vilven, R.D., California State University
Director of Pritikin Systems, Inc.

THE NEW
PRITIKIN™
PROGRAM

*The easy and delicious way to shed fat,
lower your cholesterol, and stay fit*

Robert Pritikin

DIRECTOR OF THE PRITIKIN LONGEVITY CENTER

SIMON AND SCHUSTER
New York   London   Toronto   Sydney   Tokyo

Simon and Schuster
Simon & Schuster Building
Rockefeller Center
1230 Avenue of the Americas
New York, New York 10020

Designed by Irving Perkins Associates
Manufactured in the United States of America

1   3   5   7   9   10   8   6   4   2

Library of Congress Cataloging-in-Publication data

Pritikin, Robert.
The new Pritikin program : the easy and delicious way to shed fat,
lower your cholesterol, and stay fit / Robert Pritikin.
p.   cm.
Includes bibliographical references (p.   )
1. Low-fat diet.   2. Physical fitness—Nutritional aspects.
I. Title.
RM237.7.P77   1990
613.2'5—dc20   89-21938
CIP

ISBN-13: 978-1-4165-8576-3 ISBN-10: 1-4165-8576-1

This book is dedicated to the memory of my father,
Nathan Pritikin.

Contents

THE NEW PRITIKIN PROGRAM

Introduction

One of my father's favorite analogies had to do with arsenic. Imagine a society, he'd say, where people were crazy about arsenic—they loved the way it tasted, and it went with just about every food. They sprinkled it on cereal, stirred it into hot drinks, cooked it into meat, vegetables, bread, desserts. Soon you couldn't buy a food that wasn't doused with arsenic: It was an unbeatable flavor-enhancer and no one could imagine food without it.

Then people started getting sick. Some people's hair fell out, others lost their teeth, others got nauseated and dizzy or suffered excruciating headaches. Some people even died, right in the middle of a golf game or after lunch! What was going on? Was there any common link in all these different illnesses?

Doctors, nutritionists, and other experts scrambled around trying to cure what seemed to be a growing number of baffling diseases. Some even wondered if it could be arsenic—it was in everything, wasn't it? But no, it couldn't be. Look at all the people who ate just as much arsenic as everyone else—and seemed to be fine!

So the Hair Association funded research into new hair-loss treatments and better hair transplants. The Tooth Association came up with "new, improved" false teeth and dental aids. Pharmaceutical companies pushed a wide range of drugs to combat nausea, dizziness, and headaches. Some of these preparations did what they claimed to do—but most had side effects that were as bad as the symptoms they were designed to alleviate! And none of them worked on every disease. You took one drug to combat this symptom, and another—or several—appeared in its place. If you took more than one drug at a time they often counteracted each other, or

15

led to completely new symptoms—everything from diarrhea to impotence!

Then came some truly terrible news: Research seemed to indicate that a common link in some of these illnesses *might*, after all, be excess arsenic. But people couldn't do without arsenic—they loved it too much! It was what made food *good*.

Drug companies, dietitians, and medical specialists fell over themselves trying to come up with solutions. "Experts" told television audiences they could "get all of the taste of arsenic and none of the harm with Product X." "Health foods" boasted things like "23 percent less arsenic per serving!" Best-selling books (*Who Says You Can't Eat Arsenic?* ran one popular title) vied in a market hungry for a quick fix—and for the taste of arsenic. In the medical establishment, the gears ground slowly: "Nothing," they reported, was "quite conclusive yet."

And still people got sick, and died. Finally, someone who'd been following all this because he was suffering so badly himself, and was frustrated because no medication seemed to help him, got an idea: "What would happen if I just *stopped* eating arsenic?" So that's exactly what he did. And what happened was remarkable—even miraculous. His symptoms disappeared. All those cures, promises, and quick fixes, all those megadoses of vitamins and minerals, all the drugs and all the medicines—suddenly he didn't need any of them. And there was a dividend: Food *didn't* need arsenic to taste good! In fact, once he stopped adding arsenic to his food, he liked it better than when it was doused in the stuff.

My father, Nathan Pritikin, liked this story because it was, in effect, his own story. His poison wasn't arsenic, of course. His—and our—poison (which he deduced from evidence so clear that it seems amazing today that nobody else was willing to draw the same conclusions from it) was excess fat, cholesterol, and salt—and foods so overprocessed that they're virtually devoid of nutrition. And just as in his story about arsenic, the symptoms of *this* "poisoning" aren't always obvious—they can crop up unpredictably, or may not appear at *all* in certain people, at least not for many years. What's worse, not only is the damage from excess fat, cholesterol, and salt sometimes silent, it's also deadly: In a good percentage of cases, the *first* symptom of heart disease is sudden death.

My father suffered from arterial blockage so severe that his doctors simply told him, "Keep your fingers crossed." But once he stopped taking "poison," he quite naturally stopped suffering that "poison's" effects! Believe it or not, that was regarded as a radical solution thirty years ago, simple as it seems now. It's also the central message of the astonishingly effective program that bears the Pritikin name: If you don't want to get poisoned, don't eat poison.

Simple as that message is, some people still resist it. Against all evidence, driven by what they're sure is an irresistible craving for foods that "taste good" (possible, of course, only if the foods are laden with fat, cholesterol, or salt), they're determined to eat poison anyway. Frankly, what I tell these people is simple, too: If you're going to add the poison of excess fat, cholesterol, and salt to your food, you might as well take all the antidotes you can. You're going to need all the help you can get.

Luckily, there's a much better alternative. Perhaps this is your first exposure to the Pritikin program. If it is, you may be surprised to hear that the claims my father made about the link between the foods we eat and their effects on coronary heart disease, high blood pressure, diabetes, and a host of other life-threatening illnesses, including certain forms of cancer, were not completely accepted by the medical establishment. However, by accumulating and disseminating irrefutable evidence—clinical results of Pritikin program followers that were first published in 1974 (since then, further results have been published in twenty-eight scientific papers), two Senate committee appearances leading to nationwide recommendations to lower fat in the diet, a citing by the American Heart Association, chapters in two medical textbooks—my father broke new ground. He established principles of health and nutrition now—finally!—increasingly advocated by the medical establishment. And, again, his main principle was simple: If you don't want to get poisoned, don't eat poison!

The Pritikin Centers across the country, and the research now being carried out by the Nathan Pritikin Research Foundation, continue to corroborate my father's first findings—findings we've made the basis of the Pritikin program. The results of staying with this program are dramatic—and they speak for themselves. The first 893 people to participate in a 26-day Pritikin Longevity Center program provided us with a wealth of data, which were then evaluated by the Department of Biostatistics and Epidemiology at Loma Linda

University.[1] Here are a few highlights, well known to some by now (many of these facts have already appeared in medical journals), but if you're new to the Pritikin program, they'll show you why we're so enthusiastic about our program:

- 83 percent of hypertensive people who entered the program on medication *lowered their blood pressure to normal and left drug-free*—even some participants who had been on drugs for many years.
- Over 50 percent of adult-onset diabetics on insulin left the program *free of insulin;* over 90 percent of diabetics on oral drugs left *free of drugs.*
- For many people suffering from angina, pain was greatly diminished, and *62 percent of drug-taking angina patients left the center drug-free,* while many others were able to reduce their medication.
- Cholesterol and triglycerides were each *lowered an average of 25 percent.*
- Overweight people *lost an average of 13 pounds* during the 26-day program.
- 70 percent of people suffering from claudication (blockage in the arteries of the legs) were greatly helped—even those with severe blockage and leg pains.
- In 1976, sixty-four people recommended for bypass surgery went through the Pritikin program instead. By 1981, *80 percent of them still had not undergone surgery.*[2]

The clearest single reason for these happy results is that our program is a *preventive* one—not a series of desperate "Band-Aid" attempts to deal with this or that symptom. By getting to the root of what causes many serious illnesses, the Pritikin program makes it largely unnecessary to search for "cures" for obesity, high blood pressure, arterial disease, and diabetes—our program gives you the best insurance you can have that you won't develop these conditions in the first place! If you *have* developed them, however, we can help you control many of them. The proof is in the statistics you just read.

And the proof is coming from *outside* the Pritikin Centers as well. In a recent test conducted at the University of California School of Medicine by Dean Ornish, M.D., severe cardiac patients who stopped smoking and followed a program of a 10 percent fat diet, moderate exercise, and stress management actually demonstrated reversal of coronary artery blockage.[3]

If the Pritikin program isn't new to you—perhaps you've even looked at some of my father's previous books—the dramatic results

I've just cited won't be news either. But you may be worried that it's difficult to follow the Pritikin plan: Isn't cutting back on fat, cholesterol, and salt, and concentrating on whole-grain foods, fresh vegetables, and fruits, just too difficult?

No! It's just that the idea of making *any* major change can be a scary one indeed. Every time we greet a new crowd of participants at our centers we meet with the same resistance to change, so through the years we've developed an approach which is so reassuring and so workable that even the hardest to convince are won over.

One of our strongest premises is that if you want to be healthy, you've got to address *all* the factors of health. This is where you may have gone wrong before—searching for the *one* magical cure-all that will fix everything. But quick fixes simply don't work in the long run. Not only do you miss the big picture, you sometimes end up trading one problem for another, possibly worse.

The recent emphasis on niacin to reduce cholesterol is a good example, because ultimately it does you a terrible disservice: By placing so much emphasis on one or two magical solutions, it unwittingly encourages you to eat and live as unhealthily as you like. "As long as I take my niacin, I *can* have that burger and shake, can't I? Niacin will just get rid of all that cholesterol and I can eat whatever I want!" Sounds too good to be true, doesn't it? Well, niacin is an effective cholesterol-lowering drug and may be necessary for some people. But it should not be used in place of diet. A megadose of anything can be a prescription for trouble, and taking large quantities of niacin to lower your cholesterol is no different. It can irritate your stomach and raise your blood sugar, for starters, and eventually bring on serious liver trouble—even hepatitis. The recommended dietary allowance for niacin is 13 to 19 milligrams a day. Yet some people take 150 times as much!

It just doesn't pay to do it that way. If you do, you're bound to create new problems, and you're apt to miss the real point: You have to look at *all* the factors of good health. Where the burger and shake are concerned, cholesterol isn't the only problem; junk foods like these are dangerously high in fat as well.

Of course, most people want to do as little as possible to stay healthy. Who doesn't want the easy way out? If someone offered you a magic pill that would wipe away all your illnesses and all your chances of developing illness, wouldn't you take it? On the strength of that craving for a quick and easy solution, we've been deluged with high-protein quick-weight-loss diets, mix-and-match food plans, programs that tell us to eat nothing but rice and grapefruit—even, a while back, a diet making liberal use of martinis. Fiber supplements, megadoses of vitamins, diet pills that block hunger or act as diuretics: If there's anything we can pop into our mouths to cure it all, we'll take it, right? We're convinced the only alternative is to deprive ourselves of the things we love best—and that's too hard to swallow. We want to have our cake and eat it, too.

On the Pritikin program, you *can* have your cake and eat it, too! That is, we've developed a nutritional plan on which you can eat virtually as much as you want of delicious foods *without* consuming dangerous amounts of cholesterol, fat, salt, and refined sugar. If you don't eat "poison" (which you won't on the Pritikin plan), you not only won't get poisoned, you won't need to scramble around for quick fixes. There won't be anything to fix!

In the course of treating over 50,000 people at our centers in the last fifteen years, we've developed an across-the-board approach not only to nutrition but also to exercise and stress management that makes my father's principles more workable than ever. If you've heard of the Pritikin program but are convinced it's too hard to implement in your daily life, get ready for some surprises.

As you'll soon see, our plan does *not* mean deprivation. It's flexible—as easily adapted to the needs of a harried parent of four kids or an overworked businessperson as it is to the lives of those enjoying or contemplating retirement. And it's comprehensive—more so than ever—with an emphasis on life-style that's just as important as the food guidelines for which we've always been known. In fact, the need for a flexible program and the importance of stress management are two of the most vital things we've learned. Our aim is simple: We want to give you the best plan for staying healthy that you can possibly have.

And I emphasize "we." The Pritikin program has attracted some of the finest medical, nutrition, exercise, and life-style specialists in the country—all of whom have contributed to the rich store of advice you'll find in the following pages. While my name is on the front of the book, the spirit and content come from scores of others, including the thousands of participants who are just as enthusiastic about the program as we are. I hope "we" very shortly includes *you.*

PART I

Fitness, Health, and Energy for a Lifetime

CHAPTER 1

The New Pritikin Program Promise

If logic were all it took, there'd be no problem. Persuading you to follow a program that would help you lose fat and maintain optimal weight, look and feel terrific, and substantially decrease your risk of heart disease and cancer would be simple. All we'd have to do is turn the Pritikin program—which has led to greater success in achieving these goals than any other nutrition and exercise plan ever devised—into a list of simple instructions, hand them out, and you'd follow them.

The result would be astonishing. The threat of America's top three killers—heart disease, cancer, and stroke—would dramatically reduce. The vast majority of people on medication for hypertension could help keep their blood pressure down through diet and exercise alone. Thousands of Type II (adult-onset) diabetics would be able to eliminate or reduce their need for medication, and thousands of others labeled "pre-diabetic" would reduce their risk of developing the disease. Virtually everyone would have the opportunity to avoid becoming overweight, because everyone would be on an eating and exercise plan that automatically enabled them to slim down and perform to potential. Calorie counting would cease, and we'd all throw out our scales. How could this possibly work, you ask? Because we'd be eating what the human organism is biologically designed to eat, and developing our bodies to their fullest potential.

If logic were all we needed, the numerous authoritative studies upon which our highly credentialed health experts have based the

23

Pritikin plan would make a central claim self-evident: A diet based on whole grains, legumes, vegetables, fruits, and limited quantities of nonfat dairy products, fish, shellfish, lean poultry, and lean red meat is what human beings thrive on. When we stick to these foods, we have a greater chance of becoming what we want to be: healthy, energetic, and fully alive, with a strong probability of a longer and more productive life.

In fact, logic *can* be persuasive—at least in the long run. Claims that Nathan Pritikin made back in 1978 in his book *The Pritikin Program for Diet and Exercise* have been validated by the same medical establishment that was reluctant to accept them ten years ago. The evidence is convincing: The principles of the Pritikin program are medically and scientifically sound. Nathan Pritikin developed an approach to nutrition that *works,* and the data that explain how and why it works are now flooding in. There's simply no doubt anymore that what we've done for most of the more than 50,000 people who have passed through our centers is what you need to do at home. If you want to lose fat, feel great, and be healthy, there's simply no better plan you can follow.

Isn't that enough? It should be, but most of us don't live by logic alone. "Doesn't this mean I'll have to give up everything that *tastes* good?" is the usual comment. "This probably works well enough, but what's life without ice cream? Or steak and fries?" Say "the Pritikin plan" to someone who's heard nothing more about it than that "they don't let you eat eggs, butter, or bacon," and he's likely to back off, wondering how anyone could ever give all that up.

Give what up? You may not have heard that we make a terrific Salmon Pâté. Great Chicken Curry. Tortilla Chips, Gazpacho, Teriyaki Steak—they're all on the menu (see the recipes in Chapter 13), as are Cranberry-Glazed Chicken Breast with Whole-Grain Stuffing, Ratatouille, Banana French Toast, Pritikin Cheesecake, and Apple-Date Cake; the list goes on and on. People on the Pritikin plan definitely eat well.

Yet scientific logic *plus* a mouth-watering menu may still not be enough. You may have decided you need to lose 10 pounds by next Tuesday, and you're tempted by the claims of the quick-fixers—"Lose 10 pounds in four days!"—which may dazzle you more than the Pritikin plan's modest-sounding 1 to 4 pounds a week. So you plunge into a short-term regimen—a high-protein quick-weight-loss diet or a handful of diuretic pills and a few sips of a liquid diet "meal"—and in a few days the scale says you've done it. Yes, you've lost some weight, but what you haven't lost is *fat:* You've lost water, and if you keep at it long enough you'll lose muscle, too. You may be able to tighten your belt a few notches temporarily, but the fluid will eventually come back—as well as more fat than you had when you started. You're worse off than ever.

Meanwhile, your next-door neighbor keeps looking better. Day after day, week after week, she's looking not only slimmer but healthier, too. Athletic—more energetic. More light in her eyes. She's down to a size 6 but she doesn't look emaciated—she looks fit. She invites you for lunch and serves (could it be?) pasta with a fresh tomato sauce, and blueberry cheesecake for dessert. How could she be losing weight if she's eating like this? You're sure she must really be starving herself every other day. But you're wrong. She's following the Pritikin plan.

The truth is she eats this well *every day,* and her body takes care of itself. She eats as much as she wants and needs, and she doesn't even bother to check her weight anymore, because she knows that as long as she sticks to a few simple principles, she'll weigh what she ought to weigh. She's learned to put the emphasis on good health, and the dividend is that she's slimmer than ever.

She's concerned about improving the quality of her life, and the length of it. Her cholesterol is down to a low-risk level, and so is her blood pressure. When she feels stress, she doesn't grab for potato chips or chocolate: She's learned far more effective ways to calm down and ride out the rough times. She's discovered that she likes aerobic exercise; in fact, she'd never give it up. And she's learned it all from the Pritikin program.

This book will teach you the same things—and more. The principles that have worked for thousands of others will work for you, too. You may have turned to this book to lose weight, or to focus on a specific health objective—perhaps you've been told your cholesterol is too high, or that you're pre-diabetic and need to make some fundamental changes in your diet. Whatever the reason, one thing is certain: You'll get more than you bargained for!

You've made the decision to find out how much you can do for yourself. Now we'll show you how easy it is to shed excess fat, maintain a healthy weight, and stay fit. We're not offering a "quick-fix diet." We're offering you a plan that really works and that you'll want to follow for a lifetime.

A POSITIVE TREND

For decades now, the approach of the Pritikin program has gone farther than any other to ensure good health and prevent or treat many serious health conditions. These include heart disease, hypertension, diabetes, obesity, and certain forms of cancer. Today, our message is increasingly backed by solid scientific research. Based on firm medical principles, it's accepted by medical doctors and nutritionists, and its dietary guidelines meet or exceed those of a growing number of highly respected health organizations.

The American Heart Association (AHA), the American Diabetes Association, the National Heart, Lung and Blood Institute, the National Cancer Institute, and the National Academy of Sciences report on Diet and Health, among others, have recently established dietary recommendations closer to those established by the Pritikin program years ago. To help support its latest position on reducing cholesterol, the AHA cited a study conducted by the Nathan Pritikin Research Foundation.[1] The AHA also acknowledged that by following an eating plan similar to ours, you can enhance your health and lower your risk factors for heart and blood-vessel disease. But while these associations are moving in the right direction, clinical trials have demonstrated our approach to be more effective in lowering cholesterol.

Nutritional recommendations from the federal government were widely publicized in former Surgeon General C. Everett Koop's first report on nutrition and disease, released in July 1988.[2] His report emphasized the connection between a diet high in fats and a heightened risk of heart disease, some cancers, diabetes, high blood pressure, strokes, and other chronic, serious conditions. This same position has always been the key principle behind the Pritikin program. The surgeon general's 712-page report urged Americans to increase their consumption of complex carbohydrates and fiber by emphasizing fresh vegetables and fruits and whole-grain foods. It also recommended that Americans "achieve and maintain a desirable body weight" through sensible eating habits and regular exercise, while reducing their intake of salt and alcohol. All of this has been at the heart of the Pritikin program since its very beginning, and now the rest of the world is embracing some of the same healthy concepts.

In November 1988, Dr. Dean Ornish of the University of California School of Medicine presented the preliminary results of his landmark study of fifty subjects with severe coronary heart disease: Ten of Ornish's first twelve patients following a program of a 10 percent fat diet, moderate exercise, stress management, and smoking cessation demonstrated *reversal* of coronary atherosclerosis, whereas eleven of the first seventeen in the control group showed measurable *worsening* of their coronary artery blockage![3] Dr. Ornish had set out to see, among other things, if a drug-free program can actually reverse arterial closure. His findings—the first clinical documentation that such reversal *is* indeed possible without using drugs, by following a program of low-fat eating, exercise, and life-style management like ours—are the ultimate validation of our work.

If you're an informed reader, you probably know about the AHA recommendations and the surgeon general's report already. It's likely that you've already heard that an eating plan rich in unrefined carbohydrates and fiber, low in fat, sodium, and cholesterol, and moderate in protein is superb preventive medicine, offering you lasting protection from many serious illnesses. But actually putting it to work in your own kitchen—making it part of your family's active life, or your own—may bring you to a dead halt. It's too much to make such sweeping changes in your diet, isn't it? You just know you'll feel deprived—how could you ever cope with *that?*

Don't worry. It's *much* easier to be healthy than you may think.

KEEPING IT SIMPLE

While the Pritikin Lifetime Eating Plan does call for your active involvement, there's no need to panic. You've already begun that active involvement just by picking up this book. Our whole program (which includes the Pritikin Lifetime Eating Plan, exercise, and stress management) is designed to be instituted simply. We'll guide you through every step with easy, realistic, workable suggestions. The Lifetime Eating Plan adapts equally well to life at home and on the job, and is ideal for full-size family menus, casual single living, creative entertaining, and traveling. And you'll find lots of ways to eat out just as pleasurably as you do now, whether the food is Chinese, Mexican, Italian, or French.

But what about exercises and stress management? Our goal is to help you create a *balanced* life-style, one in which each of the elements—what you eat, how you exercise, how you react to the ups and downs of daily life—complements and supports the others. If you're new to exercising, that's okay. You can take up walking, or choose from a variety of other exercises. Anyone who's made the commitment to exercise regularly and has begun to feel its benefit (which you feel in your first week) is usually horrified at the thought of ever giving it up.

Stress is such a key factor in overall health (chronic stress is linked to a whole range of diseases, from ulcers to heart attacks) that managing it is every bit as important as carefully choosing the food you eat or exercising regularly. To that end, you'll learn what stress really is, and how to recognize the signs that perhaps you're experiencing more (or, believe it or not, in a few cases, *less*) stress than is right for you. It's a lot easier than you might think to put things in balance—and once they are, not only will you want to stick to the Pritikin program, it will be far easier to.

In short, you have a vested interest in taking loving care of yourself, and making that care as thorough as it can be ensures that you'll address all the risk factors you face. Because there simply aren't any magical quick fixes for attaining and maintaining good health, the whole point of the Pritikin program is to be good to yourself *across the board.* To do that effectively, you have to lay some groundwork: Set yourself up for success! Stock your cabinets and refrigerator beforehand, so when you're exhausted after a particularly grueling day and all you know is "I'm hungry!" you'll be able to reach for something good to eat to satisfy that hunger. Prepare physically by sticking to one of the best energizers and antidepressants we know: regular exercise. And prepare emotionally by taking some time to relax (there's a great simple relaxation exercise in Chapter 17—it's a wonderful way to start or end each day).

IMPROVEMENT ACROSS THE BOARD

Jeff G., who reduced his cholesterol level by over one-half *and* lost 35 pounds in less than four months, sums up his own experience as a follower of the Pritikin program: "Through the program, I learned that what I eat regularly has a direct effect on how I look and feel, and on my sense of well-being," he says. "I just never realized how much *choice* I had to feel better. As I see how making the right choices pays off, I'm learning to make them again and again, every day. It's as if I get up each morning and renew a pact with myself— let's see how good I can make it for myself today!" Jeff says that the emphasis on eating nourishing, creative, but easy-to-prepare meals and on staying active brings some surprising rewards. "Not only am I lightening up physically, I'm lightening up emotionally. My energy level is on a steady high—no more huge swoops of mood and fatigue—and I feel as good inside as I look outside."

After years on the standard American diet, you probably don't know what it feels like to be at your mental and physical peak. (You've got a wonderful surprise coming!) Feeling lethargic or stressed out is to most people the simple consequence of a normal day's routine. We accept that we're exhausted by 7:30 at night— that's just the way it is. We're taught, and we teach ourselves, to accept less than an optimal state of health because we don't know any better. It's no wonder, then, that alumni of the Pritikin program invariably report being surprised at how terrific they feel after just several weeks on the program. Most say they are more energetic, vigorous, and alert—as well as leaner—than they've been for many years.

Overall improvement is virtually standard for followers of the Pritikin program. Listen to Diane L., a thirty-four-year-old department-store buyer who came to us complaining of frequent fatigue. Thirty pounds overweight, she had a total cholesterol level of 260 milligrams per deciliter (mg/dl), which, as you'll learn later, is dangerously high; she suffered from recurrent headaches and never slept very well. Heart disease and hypertension ran in her family, and she feared that she was increasingly at risk, but felt that many of her health problems were inevitable, beyond her control.

"When I first found out about the Pritikin program," she says, "I was skeptical. For one thing, I had been on many diets before, most of them the high-protein type, and I wasn't so sure that switching to meals high in carbohydrates would help me lose weight. Eating pasta to lose weight sounded like a big contradiction!" Neither could Diane imagine how just changing her eating and exercise habits could take care of her other medical problems, but she'd tried everything else, so she finally came to us. And faster than she ever dreamed, her health was transformed. After just eight weeks, she not only lost most of her extra weight, but also saw her blood cholesterol drop nearly 80 points. She found she had a great deal of energy left after a long working day. Her headaches disappeared, her sleep improved, and even her blood pressure showed a moderate decline.

"I had lost weight before," Diane explains, "but I always gained it back and I never had enough energy. I just assumed that feeling this way was the norm, considering my demanding job and my bad family history." At first, Diane couldn't believe that the Pritikin plan was encouraging her to eat things like fresh roasted potatoes, pasta primavera, crusty whole-grain bread, and hearty cereals—all the starchy foods she loved. But Diane learned quickly that by eating meals abundant in all kinds of unrefined carbohydrates and low in fat and cholesterol, she almost couldn't help losing weight and feeling terrific. Her extra pounds steadily dropped away, along with her risk factors for major diseases—the double dividend that distinguishes the Pritikin Lifetime Eating Plan from all others.

A PROGRAM FOR EVERYONE

What if you already look lean and fit? Is the Pritikin program for you, too? Aren't you automatically protected from most diseases if you've kept your weight down and you work out at the gym?

Unfortunately, just as you can't judge a book by its cover, you can't judge a person's health by how much body fat he or she has. It's perfectly possible to look like—or even *be*—a marathon runner, and collapse suddenly from a stroke or heart attack. "Normal" body weight is no shield from serious illness, and it may give you a false sense of security. People who are developing heart disease, hypertension, diabetes, and other ills rarely show any obvious symptoms, and in fact may seem perfectly healthy until a full-blown problem emerges.

The media are no help. One commercial for a California health club features a slim, beautiful actress who confesses to eating junk food all day long—then adds quickly that it's okay since she "burns it all off" by exercising. Exercise will certainly promote the loss of excess body fat, particularly when combined with the right eating plan. And it can help (as you'll learn) by raising your level of HDL (or "good") cholesterol a modest degree. However, it's far more possible—and far more important—to lower your LDL (or "bad") cholesterol level, and thereby your total cholesterol, something best accomplished by following a low-fat diet.

You just can't "burn off" the cholesterol you eat, no matter how hard you work out. Some wiry long-distance runners—seemingly the healthiest, fittest people around—have died of "silent" heart disease at an early age. Even the most vigorous exercise couldn't save them from the ultimate consequences of an unhealthy life-style (such as eating habits or smoking habits). Thin and physically fit do not automatically mean healthy. Only a sound program, including the Pritikin Lifetime Eating Plan, can help you to be all three.

NATURAL WEIGHT LOSS

If you're like the majority of people who come to our Pritikin Centers, your problem isn't that you're "wiry." The mirror tells you you've got to lose weight. Now there's nothing wrong with a good healthy dose of vanity—of course you want to look terrific! So, if excess weight has gotten you to these pages, just as it gets so many people into our health centers, fine. You can expect to lose all that fat, simply and steadily. As we've seen with our friend Diane L., becoming slimmer is the lifetime *bonus* of the Pritikin plan—a dividend of following a program that's geared to make you fit and healthy.

The principles of healthy eating that form our eating plan apply to everyone, those who need to lose weight as well as those who don't. But if you're interested in a faster rate of weight loss than that which would occur naturally over a longer period of time, or if you've got an especially severe weight problem, you can still follow the Lifetime Eating Plan, but with some easy modifications, to reach your goal a bit more quickly.

Today's average American menu derives about 35 to 45 percent of its total calories from fat, 10 to 15 percent from protein, and 40 to 45 percent from (mostly refined) carbohydrates. By contrast, the meals on the slimming, health-enhancing Pritikin Lifetime Eating Plan derive up to 10 percent of their total calories from fat, 10 to 15 percent from protein, and about 75 to 80 percent from carbohydrates, mostly complex and unrefined.

While the percentage of protein on the American and Pritikin eating plans is similar, the source is not. On the Pritikin eating plan, most of the protein comes from nonfat dairy foods and low-fat, high-fiber plant foods—grains, vegetables, legumes, and fruits in their whole or nearly natural form, the same foods that are rich in beneficial unrefined carbohydrates. The standard American diet, however, gets most of its protein from fatty, cholesterol-rich animal sources. As you'll see in Chapter 7, this difference turns out to be crucial.

The Pritikin Lifetime Eating Plan promotes weight loss in a variety of ways. The largely unrefined carbohydrate foods you'll eat are lower in calories and naturally filling; the lean animal protein, which comes from fish, lean poultry, and lean red meat (such as flank and round steak), is relatively low in fat; the dairy foods are nonfat; and the dishes are seasoned with a variety of delicious spices—with little or no added salt or sugar (you won't miss them!). Such a low-fat, high-carbohydrate eating plan automatically aids in trimming pounds away: Because it takes less energy to store excess dietary fat as body fat than it does to store excess carbohydrates as body fat, the dietary fat you eat is far more likely to turn into excess body fat. That simply can't happen on the Pritikin plan.

What's more, this plan will change your eating patterns and tastes—encouraging you, perhaps, to eat more frequently throughout the day (pick-me-up snacks between meals), and opening up a wonderful new world of flavor for you to enjoy. People who give up excess fat soon discover they don't miss it, and eventually grow to dislike even the thought of eating it! Yes, it's true that fat is a flavor enhancer, but when we cut it out of our diet, the true flavors of other foods come through and become enormously appealing. You'll discover that the taste of whole-grain rye bread is wonderful—without butter. And that you haven't really eaten corn on the cob until you've had it sweet and fresh and undoctored by butter or salt.

The Pritikin Lifetime Eating Plan is full of innovative new recipes and complete menus to get you started, plus tips to help you stockpile the right foods so you won't be tempted to grab an unhealthy snack. You can enjoy your transition to sound nutrition and better health more easily than you ever dreamed possible. If what you want is weight loss, by following the Pritikin program not only will you succeed in losing unwanted fat, you'll lower your cholesterol and blood pressure and guard against life-threatening disease as well. On the other hand, if you've turned to the Pritikin program to guard against heart disease or diabetes, you'll probably become leaner as a *dividend!* As we said earlier, you'll get more than you bargained for.

WHY THE PROGRAM WORKS

The Pritikin program works because it addresses *every* manageable health factor you face: It not only offers proven eating and exercise plans, but it will change the way you *look* at yourself. By learning new strategies to reclaim your health and energy, you'll feel a new power to affect the course of your life: The program will work, ultimately, because you'll want it to work! It's not that there won't be occasional stumbling blocks or moments when you'll have doubts, but we'll help you anticipate those blocks and help you get through them. Nobody's perfect, and almost everyone suffers a lapse now and then. If you get off track, we'll show you how to get back on.

Above all, we hope you'll soon become conscious of what you eat, what it tastes like, and what you're doing to help or hinder your health. Our first goal is to show you that you do have a choice, that there are many things you can do right now to start getting healthy. Self-deprivation isn't our watchword—self-awareness is.

This book is divided into three parts. In Part I you'll learn the basics of the soundest eating plan there is, and how a program of healthy eating, sensible exercise, and stress management can help you lose unwanted fat, transform the way you feel, reduce your risk for life-threatening disease, and quite possibly add years to your life as well.

Part II is an up-to-date rundown of all the nutrition and health information you'll need. Here you'll get the most recent findings on carbohydrates, fiber, fat, cholesterol, protein, and sodium, and learn how each promotes or undermines your health and weight-loss goals.

All the things you've been wondering about (What *is* the difference between fat and cholesterol, anyway? How important *is* fiber in my diet? What's the real scoop on protein?) will be addressed. We'll sort out confusing health claims, separate fact from myth, and summarize all the latest scientific and nutrition information that forms the basis for the practical recommendations we'll give you next.

In Part III you'll find our entire eating, exercise, weight-loss, and stress-reduction program. There are dozens of exciting recipes here, ideas for healthful cooking and menu planning, and guidelines for eating out. You'll learn how to eat well at parties, on the road—or even abroad! Best of all, this section is complete with easy ways to *make it work*, including techniques to help you achieve your goals, whatever they are.

This combination of everyday advice and current research makes the Pritikin Lifetime Eating Plan a realistic and reassuring one: It will help you cope with a variety of hard-to-avoid temptations and teach you how to choose the very best alternatives under less than ideal conditions. With the facts as your guide, you'll learn how to minimize your health risks and choose sensibly in mealtime situations that are beyond your control.

So, what are we offering you? A simple eating plan for weight loss and weight maintenance. A proven plan for dramatically decreasing your risk of cardiovascular disease and many kinds of cancer, as well as guarding against diabetes. An across-the-board approach that addresses *all* the life-style-related risk factors of life-threatening disease—not just one. An exercise plan you can implement simply and quickly. A perspective that provides you with the power to make strong, positive changes in every area of your life and health. Food that's not only good for you but tastes terrific. And the knowledge of how all of this works together to promise you the best health and the longest, most productive life you can have.

You've already taken advantage of this abundance, simply by opening this book. Now let us show you how much more you can do! It's the best investment of time and energy you can possibly make: You're handing yourself a whole new life.

CHAPTER 2

Beyond Dieting: The Pritikin Lifetime Eating Plan

If you're like most people, you approach the food guidelines in most diet books with a good deal of apprehension. We've been besieged by so many books that blithely tell us (in effect) to rip apart our kitchen cupboards and refrigerators and throw everything out— then eat nothing but grapefruit (or rice or carrot sticks or hamburger). Seldom is our sense of comfort more threatened than when some "expert" charges in and tells us to stop eating all the things we love.

Unfortunately, the Pritikin Lifetime Eating Plan was once accused of not appealing enough to the taste buds. Ironically, it was Nathan Pritikin's own zeal that sometimes overshadowed the message that you *can* enjoy food that's good for you: "Basically," he once said, "all I'm trying to do is wipe out heart disease, hypertension, and diabetes in this country." In fact, we *will* ask you to rethink what you eat, but we guarantee you'll be surprised by how much we'll encourage you to continue eating foods you already enjoy.

As for discarding what *isn't* good for you, one follower of the Pritikin program says, "Whenever I come across another forgotten can of salty, fatty soup, I remember how amazed my doctor was when he saw my blood pressure go down just from changing my diet. I find new courage to say no." By focusing on all the foods you *can* eat, as well as on the pleasure of eating the ones you love most

35

(like baked potatoes, or corn on the cob, or pasta cooked al dente with tomatoes, garlic, and basil), you begin to set yourself up for real health success.

One thing you'll hear frequently from us: *Focus on your goals.* Not with blinders—not grimly, expecting deprivation—but with *optimism.* The kind of optimism that comes from knowing that you're keeping your blood pressure and cholesterol at safe levels; providing yourself with plenty of fiber, vitamins, and other nutrients; and following the most effective long-term weight-loss and -maintenance program ever offered.

And while health always comes first with the Pritikin program, enjoyment is a simultaneous dividend. We know from our own experience, both firsthand and from the tens of thousands of people who've passed through our centers and followed our Lifetime Eating Plan, that you just won't do something you don't enjoy. But if you take a new look at all the foods we have to offer, you won't need a pep talk. You'll quickly see the benefits—in health and taste—for yourself.

BEYOND DIETING

What do we mean when we say the Pritikin Lifetime Eating Plan isn't a diet? It's not a "diet" quite simply because it's not temporary; it isn't something you "do" for a few weeks when you feel you need to shed a few pounds. We offer something that goes far beyond diets you may have encountered before. Our Pritikin plan enables you to revamp your *whole* approach to food—to make an across-the-board difference in your health.

Making that kind of change isn't always easy. It's especially hard when you're reluctant to face up to health risks you know you face. When you *know* your blood pressure or cholesterol level is too high, when you *know* you've got to lose 20 pounds, but you deny that it's all *that* serious. That denial is dangerous—especially in the case of heart disease, where you often don't have a clue until it's virtually too late. People who experience no pain or any other outward warning symptoms whatsoever, people who are overweight but eat too much cholesterol, fat, salt, and sugar anyway (and don't especially care because they *feel* all right)—they're also the people who may suddenly have a stroke or heart attack. Cardiovascular disease is the number-one killer in the United States today—and a largely silent one.

Glenn D. recalls that it took his wife five years to persuade him that both of them should start the Pritikin program. Glenn was overweight and out of shape—230 pounds, with a cholesterol level that hovered around 265 mg/dl. "But I felt okay," he says. "Numbers didn't mean much to me." Glenn's denial was further bolstered by his expressed desire to "live life to the fullest. So what if I shaved off a year or two? Life wasn't worth it if I couldn't do exactly what I wanted. To me, a good life meant as much steak and ice cream as I could keep down." His wife, Madeline, 20 pounds overweight, thought she was more enlightened: She'd given up red meat and was virtually vegetarian—which meant plenty of whole milk, cheese, eggs, and butter, and a cholesterol level of 243.

But when their close friend Phil dropped dead of a heart attack, Glenn finally woke up. Phil was about his age—forty-five—and had the same motto: Live for today—who cares about tomorrow? Suddenly, the idea of dying as a result of bad health habits didn't seem so abstract to Glenn, and "life" began to mean more than just another rich meal. So when Glenn and Madeline finally arrived at the Pritikin Center, they had already begun to understand how the wrong food can quite literally kill you.

Today, Glenn is a trim, muscular 170 pounds with a cholesterol level of 156. Madeline is now down to a trim 125 and her cholesterol has dropped to 140. Neither can quite believe what's happened to them. "Life can still be a banquet without excess salt, sugar, or fat," says Madeline. "And now we've got a good chance of staying around a long time to enjoy it!" Not only did Madeline and Glenn achieve their initial weight-loss goals, they discovered new reserves of energy—a sense of vigor and well-being they'd never known before. Says Glenn, "Living life to the fullest is just the opposite of what I thought it was."

MULTIPLE REWARDS

If someone told you that after just four weeks of eating delicious foods—five or six times a day—you would begin to look and feel better than you had in years, lose excess body fat (and weight), and cut your cholesterol by an average of 25 percent, wouldn't you be a little suspicious? After all, America's bookshelves—and very likely your own—are tumbling over with best-sellers that claim short-order miracles. As you know (probably from a good deal of firsthand experience), not only do most of these purveyors of weight-loss hype not work in the long run, but they're often hazardous to your health as well.

But there isn't one suggestion we make in our eating plan that hasn't been assiduously and authoritatively backed up. Which means you can trust this medically sound general claim: *By following the Pritikin program, it is possible that after a very short time you will—if you want to—lose fat and weight (1 to 3 pounds a week for women, 2 to 4 pounds a week for men), note a marked decrease in elevated blood pressure and serum cholesterol, and see a marked increase in endurance and energy. Plus, there's a good chance you'll look and feel better.*

One young woman from France, Marie L., who'd tried any number of "spa treatments" in Europe to help her lose weight, had become so demoralized that she'd begun to spend most of her time sleeping—sometimes sixteen hours a day. She was just about to give up when her mother discovered the Pritikin program and convinced Marie to go to a Pritikin Center. Only a month later, at Marie's eager insistence, her mother traveled across the Atlantic to visit. At the airport she cried when she saw her transformed daughter: "She was quite simply a different person—so much slimmer, lighter on her feet, and *happier.*" It's moving to see the kind of transformation the Pritikin program can effect: Marie lost weight, and gained self-esteem. She finally realized she had the *power* to transform herself—a power she could exercise most simply and effectively by following the Pritikin program.

Marie and everyone else we've helped to achieve weight loss and health goals realized that in taking on the Pritikin program, they were making a commitment, not so much to the "program" as to themselves. As we've said before, you'll never stay with something you don't want to do—but you'll *want* to follow the Pritikin program because its rewards are so great. The health benefits kick in right away and simply get better as you go on. And since the pleasure of staying with it is so considerable—the taste and satisfaction of the good food you eat—you've got further inducement to renew your pact with yourself every day. As we've said, the Pritikin Lifetime Eating Plan is a way of life, not a diet.

It's an approach that will enable you to shed excess pounds without chronic hunger, even if weight loss is not your primary goal. Jack G., a man whose blood pressure hovered around 170/110 when he came to us, had no trouble realizing he had to do something immediately to put himself at less risk for a heart attack. He was surprised to see himself in the mirror after a few weeks on the Pritikin plan: "You mean I get to *look* good, too?" he exclaimed. His blood pressure came down, to 120/80, and so did his weight, and he wasn't even trying!

Weight loss takes care of itself because the plan's mainstays are naturally filling, highly nutritious foods low in fat and high in fiber—ideally slimming choices. Because they contain so little fat, you can eat satisfying amounts of them and still lose unwanted body fat without the tedium of calorie counting or monotonous, unimaginative meals. The bottom line? You'll never feel either hungry or deprived on this plan. And in no time you'll know this is the plan to sustain for a lifetime. As one woman says, "I've got so much energy now and I look forward to every meal—why would I ever want to stop? I used to feel guilty every time I put something in my mouth; now I congratulate myself!"

WHAT EXACTLY IS THE PRITIKIN LIFETIME EATING PLAN?

The Pritikin Lifetime Eating Plan is exactly what it says it is: a design for lifelong nutrition. It provides all the nutrients you need and emphasizes foods as they are grown: fruits and vegetables; whole grains and cereals; beans, peas, and potatoes. It also features modest amounts of nonfat (not low-fat) dairy foods, as well as fish, lean poultry, and lean red meat.

You can already see from that list that the Pritikin plan includes all the familiar foods you already eat. What makes it different?

For starters, the typical American diet is shockingly high in fat, cholesterol, and sodium, and moderate in complex carbohydrates and fiber. It is also too high in nutritionally empty calories—namely, refined oils and refined sugars. By contrast, the meals on the Pritikin Lifetime Eating Plan are low in total fat (especially saturated fat), cholesterol, and sodium, and rich in unrefined carbohydrates, vitamins, minerals, and dietary fiber.

TABLE 2-1
AMOUNTS OF FOOD COMPONENTS CONSUMED ON TWO EATING PLANS

	Pritikin Lifetime Eating Plan	Standard American Diet
Fat, % of calories/day	10 or less	35–45
Protein, % of calories/day	10–15	10–15
Carbohydrates, % of calories/day	75–80	40–45
Cholesterol, mg/day	100 or less	450–500
Fiber, g/day	35 or more	10–15
Sodium, mg/day	1,600 or less	3,500–6,500

The figures in Table 2-1 show the dramatic difference between the recommendations of the Pritikin Lifetime Eating Plan and the standard American diet. You'll see that while the categories are the same, the *percentages* (for all but protein) are quite different. The Pritikin plan derives most of its protein from low-fat animal foods (nonfat dairy items and lower-fat meats) and nonanimal sources (grains, vegetables, legumes, and fruits), not the high-fat meats and dairy foods of the typical American diet. But don't be concerned—you'll still be getting more than enough protein from these healthy sources. (If you need to be convinced, read Chapter 7—it's an eye-opener!)

It's these dramatically different percentages—and the different sources of protein, carbohydrates, and other nutrients—that account for the Lifetime Eating Plan's phenomenal success. Most people who follow it will lower their serum cholesterol level to our recommendation of 160 mg/dl—or 100 mg/dl plus your age (but not to exceed 160). You're also likely to modify other risk factors for heart and blood-vessel disease, as well as decrease your chances of developing hypertension, diabetes, obesity, and certain forms of cancer, such as breast and colon cancer.

ANOTHER LIFETIME BONUS: TOP NUTRITION

The foods on the Pritikin plan—low in fat, high in fiber, and moderate in protein—not only will reduce your risk for major diseases and help you lose weight, but will also fulfill all your nutritional needs. A recent study was conducted to establish the long-term nutritional adequacy of the Pritikin Lifetime Eating Plan. In over forty blood tests, we found no signs of any inadequacy in the levels of vitamins, minerals, protein, and iron.[1] The subjects tested had not taken vitamin or mineral supplements. This isn't surprising, since the Pritikin plan exceeds the recommended dietary allowances for vitamins and minerals.

In the study, twenty people who followed the Lifetime Eating Plan for more than four years were compared with twenty controls who followed the standard American diet. Total cholesterol and LDL cholesterol were significantly lower in the group following the Pritikin plan; in fact, cholesterol averaged 160 mg/dl (compared to 241 mg/dl in the age-matched control group)—and 160 mg/dl is a level that virtually eliminates blood cholesterol as a risk factor for coronary heart disease! There were no significant differences between the two groups in blood levels of protein, phosphorus, calcium, magnesium, zinc, copper, or iron (in fact, one woman in the American diet group turned out to be iron deficient). The same was true for vitamins B_2, B_6, and B_{12}. What's more, those on the Pritikin plan showed higher serum levels of vitamins A and B_1. Such evidence strongly suggests that the Pritikin plan can control your cholesterol, blood sugar, lipids (blood fats), blood pressure, and body weight while maintaining safe and adequate amounts of all essential vitamins, minerals, and other nutrients!

In fact, most Americans (except, perhaps, for the elderly) need to care more about the risks of obtaining too *much* from their diets rather than too little—overdosing on vitamins to the point of toxicity as well as eating too much cholesterol, fat, and salt. Where nutrition is concerned, too much is indeed too much!

GO, CAUTION, AND STOP

Perhaps the biggest advance we've made in enhancing the livability of the Pritikin plan is to give you choices, and we've devised a simple system to help you make the best ones possible. We know it's sometimes difficult to follow an ideal eating plan when you eat at a restaurant or coffee shop, when you travel, or when you're invited to a party—so we've made room for that. We recognize that you must find *your* own level of commitment to a plan we know will work for you, and you don't have to be perfect to derive significant benefits from the Pritikin plan.

"What amazes me," one graduate student and amateur athlete told us, "is how much easier it is to eat healthy foods when I'm not at home than I thought it would be. Sometimes it's a challenge, but I look on it as a game—one that I usually end up winning!"

We group all food selections into three broad categories: "Go," "Caution," and "Stop." Here's a brief introduction to these groups.

"Go" foods, as you've no doubt already figured out, are the healthiest, most nutritious ones. The meal plans and recipes we've put together—like the ones you'll want to follow—are all based on this abundant group of delicious foods. "Caution" foods, eaten in limited amounts, probably won't have too adverse an effect, although they aren't recommended. And, of course, anything labeled "Stop" means just that! These are the foods and beverages high in fat, cholesterol, sodium, and caffeine that can be damaging to your health—even if consumed in small quantities.

You'll learn more about these different categories and what foods they contain in Chapter 11. Then you'll quickly become a pro at identifying those foods which are best for you, and at using them to create deliciously healthful meals that are low in fat and cholesterol and high in unrefined carbohydrates.

THE PRITIKIN PROGRAM'S WEIGHT-LOSS ADVANTAGE

Most people who need to lose weight will do so simply by following the Pritikin Lifetime Eating Plan. The even more pleasant surprise is that most people can lose weight on 1,500 or more calories a day—because (as you'll learn later on) your body naturally burns most of what you eat on the Pritikin plan. However, if you want to lose weight as quickly as possible, you can easily limit your caloric intake on the Pritikin plan and still not go hungry. A version of the Lifetime Eating Plan based on a minimum of 1,000 calories a day for women and 1,200 calories a day for men offers maximal weight loss, and the three weeks of creative menus featured in Chapter 13 cover both calorie levels.

Why *minimums?* A 1,000-calorie intake for women and a 1,200-

calorie intake for men are the lowest levels that can reasonably ensure an adequate supply of all nutrients and also preserve lean body tissue. Once you lose your desired weight on the 1,000- to 1,200-calorie menus you can simply step up the quantity of foods you're already eating. There's no question of shifting to a new plan—you're already on it! That's another reason the Pritikin eating plan works psychologically: You don't have to depart from it to "go on a diet." It works equally well to help you lose weight or to help you maintain your ideal weight.

Evidence suggests that the body responds to caloric intakes below 1,000 a day as if it were in a state of semi-starvation: Your body may adapt to being deprived by efficiently burning calories more slowly. Moreover, on typical crash diets, which don't provide adequate energy from carbohydrates, the human body begins to consume its own lean muscle as well as fat.

But the Pritikin plan won't assault your body the way crash diets do. A low-fat diet high in unrefined carbohydrates and fiber enables you to reach your ideal weight by shedding pounds gradually but steadily. Such moderate, natural weight loss occurs without hunger as your body adapts to a more natural fuel. You won't feel starved and your body won't overreact by radically conserving calories. What's more, by providing both adequate calories and an abundance of carbohydrates, the Pritikin Lifetime Eating Plan will keep the loss of lean muscle to a minimum while eliminating excess body fat.

A COMPLETE PROGRAM—FOR A LIFETIME

We know this may sound like a hyped-up testimonial, but the fact is that the food is so enjoyable and the improvement so dramatic, the Pritikin program can seem too good to be true!

Three meals a day, and snacks in between—all satisfying, appetizing, and good for you as well. An exercise program made just for you, and effective techniques for dealing with the stresses and challenges in your life. The almost certain result? Dramatically improved health, weight loss, more energy, and looking and feeling terrific! This is a program you'll want to stay with for your lifetime. And that could turn out to be longer than you think. Read on, and you'll learn about what may be the ultimate bonus of the Pritikin program—longevity.

CHAPTER 3

The Longevity Bonus

Will the Pritikin program give you a longer life? If diet and exercise play any role in how long you live, then the Pritikin program is one you can depend on for your best chance of living a long, productive, and enjoyable life.

With cardiovascular disease the number-one killer in America, and with most heart attacks and strokes stemming directly or indirectly from bad food habits, clearly you'll be way ahead of the game if you follow an eating plan that's low in fat and cholesterol and rich in unrefined carbohydrates. And with its potential to guard against certain forms of cancer such as breast and colon and to prevent or lessen the damaging effects of diabetes, the Pritikin Lifetime Eating Plan also addresses two other big threats to longevity today.

Because the term "longevity" is officially linked with the Pritikin program, we owe it to you to explain what we mean by it—and to be specific about the ways we hope the Pritikin plan will lengthen your own life.

We believe that an overwhelming amount of scientific research as well as the medical histories of the thousands of people who've successfully recovered from heart disease and other life-threatening conditions that their doctors had once pronounced incurable give us the authority to say that you'll be much better off physically if you follow the Pritikin program.

Of course, no one can make guarantees about longevity. But to the degree that we do have control over our own health destinies—and it now appears that the degree is greater than anyone ever

44

realized—the Pritikin program shows how to play the hands we've been dealt to the best advantage, and how to improve the quality of our lives at the same time.

LIFE SPAN VERSUS LIFE EXPECTANCY

Maximal life span and life expectancy—they sound pretty much the same, but they aren't. The first refers simply to the longest period of time any individual in a given species has ever been proven to live. Each species has its own characteristic maximal life span. For humans, according to the most reliable records, this figure is about 113 years.[1] By contrast, life expectancy tells how many years, on average, we can be expected to live. In the United States, for example, the average newborn baby statistically can currently expect to live somewhere into his or her mid-seventies (although, in this country, women live an average of about four years longer than men).

Can the way you eat have a major impact on your achieving that maximal life span? One of the earliest experiments linking nutrition to longevity comes from the work of Dr. Clive McCay at Cornell University in the late 1930s. He took a group of newly weaned rats and fed them a special diet which was more than adequate nutritionally in terms of vitamins, minerals, and proteins, but was low in total calories. While this caloric deficit slowed down their usual growth rate, it nearly doubled their maximal life span![2]

Since that first pioneering effort, many other laboratory studies performed on a variety of animals have achieved similar results. Biologists now know that a moderate reduction in caloric intake over a long period of time can extend the maximal life span of laboratory animals ranging from insects to mammals. And since research on humans has shown that caloric intake drops dramatically when people switch to a low-fat, high-fiber diet,[3] it may be possible to extend *our* maximal life span as well simply by changing the way we eat.

DIET VERSUS DISEASE

As you can see, there's quite a discrepancy between life expectancy and maximal life span—the average American is, in fact, falling short of that upper limit of maximal life span by thirty or more years. Why? Although all the answers to this question are not yet fully known, the discrepancy is due both to genetic factors and to those degenerative diseases whose names are painfully familiar to us: heart and blood-vessel disease, hypertension, adult-onset diabetes, obesity, and cancer of the breast, lung, colon, or prostate—the very illnesses that have the power to shorten your life. But because the Pritikin program helps to stave off these major killers, *it* has the potential to extend your life! Here's how:

The Lifetime Eating Plan derives the vast majority of its calories from foods rich in unrefined carbohydrates, and is low in total fat, saturated fat, salt, and cholesterol—thereby reducing the risk of fatal atherosclerotic diseases such as heart attack and stroke. It's also a useful approach for regulating blood sugar (glucose) and insulin levels in both diabetics and nondiabetics, including hypoglycemics. Because it's so low in fat and naturally abundant in fiber, and is complemented by a program of regular aerobic exercise, the Pritikin plan is the best "treatment" for obesity and for the maintenance of ideal body weight.

Since recent evidence strongly links high-fat diets to a greater risk of colon, breast, and prostate cancer, following the Pritikin Lifetime Eating Plan may protect against these life-threatening diseases as well. In addition, its low-fat, low-salt, and rich potassium content certainly helps prevent hypertension. The Pritikin program also alleviates high blood pressure by promoting the loss of excess body fat, encouraging regular aerobic exercise, and limiting alcohol intake.

While refined carbohydrates are associated with weight gain and obesity (in large part because they are often found in high-fat foods), the unrefined kinds have just the opposite effect, because, with few calories, they add bulk to foods. And the fiber they contain may itself protect against a variety of digestive diseases, including colon cancer.

Here's more evidence about a dietary link to cancer, this time regarding protein: There may be some correlation, independent of fat, between a high intake of animal protein and cancers of the breast, colon, rectum, prostate, endometrium, pancreas, and kidney. In certain tests performed on laboratory animals, the ability of various substances to induce cancer in these animals seemed to be enhanced when the animals ate two or three times as much protein as they would normally require for optimal growth and development. But when the animals were given less protein than they needed for optimal growth, the cancer-inducing effects were diminished. Certainly this cannot justify a drastic lowering of *our* protein consumption, but the researchers who conducted these experiments maintain that the *source* of our protein intake should definitely be changed to favor vegetables and grains over meats and dairy foods—which is, of course, exactly the approach of the Pritikin program.[4]

Sometimes the things that are added to foods (and not the foods themselves) can be of questionable value to your health. But on the Pritikin Lifetime Eating Plan, you'll be eating foods in as close to their natural state as possible and thereby minimizing your exposure to possibly hazardous chemicals. And by following a diet based on a wide variety of mostly unrefined foods, you'll be consuming few of the countless synthetic additives that inevitably accompany processed items.

THE FREE-RADICAL CONNECTION

One other reason that the Lifetime Eating Plan may prevent a wide range of chronic diseases and promote longevity could be that it's a rich source of certain nutrients that counteract the destructive effects of oxygen within the body. While it's natural to associate oxygen with life and survival, it may actually be a harmful agent when it interacts with certain chemicals—such as the polyunsaturated fats (lipids) in our bodies, which are derived from the highly polyunsaturated oils found in the American diet.

These polyunsaturates can become very unstable in the presence of oxygen and produce powerful and potentially damaging molecules known as "free radicals." The injury these substances can inflict on the outer membranes and internal structures of human cells is random and widespread. Chronic free-radical damage is believed to accelerate aging, and many scientists consider it one of the primary factors responsible for the normal aging process itself.

Of course, if you follow the Lifetime Eating Plan, which does not include excessive polyunsaturated fatty acids—one of the primary sources of free radicals—you'll be at a distinct advantage. In addition, some of the nutrients you will consume in abundance every day on the Pritikin plan—namely, vitamins C and E, beta-carotene, and the trace mineral selenium—possess potent antioxidant properties. This means they can prevent or even neutralize the oxygen-fueled generation of free radicals from substances such as polyunsaturated fatty acids.

Many advocates of food supplements claim that taking megadoses of these antioxidant nutrients will protect your body from cellular damage and promote longevity. But there is no animal or other evidence to show that antioxidant supplements increase the likelihood of achieving a maximal life span. Since free radicals are derived from polyunsaturates, the safest way to keep your cells healthy and intact is to avoid excessive polyunsaturated fats to begin with.

It's far wiser to follow the old adage "An ounce of prevention is worth a pound of cure" than to consume large amounts of unhealthy foods and then try to counteract their ill effects with unnaturally high doses of antioxidants. If you minimize your intake of highly polyunsaturated oils, the normal amounts of vitamins C and E, beta-carotene, and selenium found in a well-selected eating plan *can* cover your body's needs and head off free-radical reactions—and there's no better way to get these nutrients than by following the Pritikin Lifetime Eating Plan. It's naturally rich in these antioxidants, since they are found largely in the whole grains and fresh vegetables and fruits that make up most of our daily menus.

BEYOND THE PHYSICAL BENEFITS

While we can't promise that you'll add a specific number of years to your life by adhering to the complete Pritikin program of healthy eating, regular exercise, and stress control, we *can* say that you'll be decreasing your health risks dramatically by following our guidelines. You'll be protected from chronic illness, your cardiovascular system will function at its peak, your endurance will be enhanced and your mood elevated. You'll have greater energy, you'll sleep better, and you'll be able to handle life's events more effectively.

And we've discovered that there's something that goes even *beyond* the physical benefits of the Pritikin plan: the positive attitude that comes from knowing you're doing all you can do to promote longevity.

It's the renewed pleasure you'll start to take in your life as you get, look, and feel better. It's the joy that comes to the man with such severe claudication (pain in the legs due to blockage of the blood vessels there) that he couldn't walk 100 yards—and then finds himself averaging six or seven miles a *week* after only several months on the Pritikin plan. It's the emotional—as well as physical—freedom that comes to the woman who's been struggling with her weight for 20 years and has now trimmed down—permanently—without going hungry and feeling run-down. There's a special light in the eyes of people on the Pritikin program that just might not have been there before—it's the glow of health, and of the pure *joy* of feeling wonderful.

Positive attitude may be hard to quantify as a component in longevity—but even if it's only a dividend of the Pritikin program, it's an invaluable gift.

We know of no better blueprint for a healthier, happier, and possibly longer life than the Pritikin program.

The rest is up to you!

PART II

The Crucial Facts

In an information-hungry society like ours, people are always anxious to know more—particularly where life-and-death matters like their own coronary health are concerned. And with all the focus on health, diet, and fitness these days, "hot" topics like fat, cholesterol, fiber, and carbohydrates are certainly on a lot of people's minds. But when faced with an avalanche of media coverage and new reports that often seem to contradict the old, some people might feel that the more they hear about these important nutritional issues, the less they understand.

While a lot of this information can seem confusing or even discouraging at first, it really doesn't have to be. First of all, a lot of it is *not* new news! At the Pritikin Centers we've been on "the cutting edge" since 1976, advocating a low-fat, low-cholesterol, high-carbohydrate eating plan and a program of sensible exercise and life-style management as the best route to optimal overall health. It's just that it's taken a while for everyone else to catch on.

But the good word is out, and people (like you!) are listening. Because you're ready to learn more, and ready to put that knowledge to use as you pursue a lifetime of new eating habits and renewed health, here's all the up-to-the-minute information you'll need on fat, cholesterol, salt, protein, fiber, and carbohydrates—all the subjects that are in the nutritional news now, and will be for some time to come!

CHAPTER 4

Facing Facts about Fat

As you'll soon learn, one of the most appealing things about the Pritikin Lifetime Eating Plan is its worry-free simplicity: an abundance of complex carbohydrates, fresh fruits, and vegetables, and just the right amount of dairy and high-protein foods. Vitamins, minerals, and fiber in perfect proportion to your body's requirements. Everything you need—and nothing that you don't.

Including excess fat! When you follow the Pritikin Lifetime Eating Plan, 10 percent of your daily calories come from fat. Because the fat that's naturally present in the foods you eat satisfies *all* your body's requirements, there's no nutritional need to add any refined fats to your diet. An average level of 10 percent of total calories from fat can easily meet your daily needs for "essential fatty acids"—and it's all there on the Lifetime Eating Plan, since some fat is found in all natural foods of vegetable (and, of course, animal) origin. In fact, the two essential fatty acids that the human body must have—linoleic acid and linolenic acid—are found in fairly generous quantities in whole grains, beans, peas, and vegetables, all mainstays of the Pritikin plan.

The small amount of dietary fat that we do need serves various functions. Fats and oils, which are made up of three fatty acids and glycerol, play a role in making up the membranes which surround all cells. These membranes hold in the cells' contents and help regulate the passage of nutrients in and out of the cells. Fatty acids are also involved in the absorption and transport of fat-soluble vitamins and cholesterol. Fats are stored for energy, and for padding and insulation for the body and its internal organs. In small amounts,

53

they're vital to growth and health—but too much of a good thing can be harmful, and this is certainly the case with fats.

THE DANGERS OF EXCESS

The fact is that we don't need nearly as much fat as most Americans consume. A mere 1 to 3 percent of our daily calories need to come from the essential fatty acids—and you'll have no problem getting these essential fatty acids on a 10 percent fat diet based on unrefined foods. Yet fat still accounts for over 35 percent of the calories in the diets of most Americans (see Figure 4-1, comparing the sources of fat in the Pritikin plan and in the American diet). And in addition to the role it plays in the obvious problem of overweight, excess dietary fat is a major predisposing factor in the development of a variety of chronic, often life-threatening diseases.

Numerous studies have shown that people around the world who don't eat excess fat very rarely get many of the serious illnesses common in America. Heart and blood-vessel disease, obesity, hypertension (except in Japan, where they eat too much salt—but we'll get

FIGURE 4-1
SOURCES OF FAT IN THE AMERICAN DIET
Based on 40% of total calories

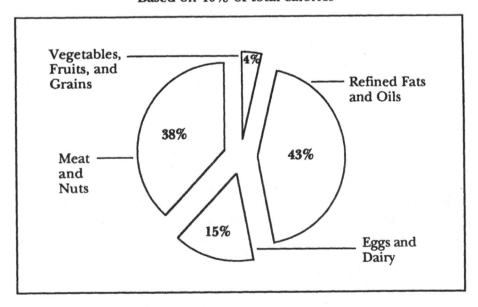

to that later), diabetes, arthritis, and certain forms of cancer are less common in populations on low-fat diets.[1] We now know that excess dietary fat can increase the risk of both breast and colon cancer, and may aggravate Type II (adult-onset) diabetes because it appears to hamper the ability of insulin to transport glucose and it promotes obesity, which is a risk factor for diabetes. Too much fat (particularly polyunsaturated fat) may increase gallstone formation. When you take a close look at percentages and amounts, you find that those who are at the lowest risk for coronary heart disease consume about 10 percent of their total calories from fat. They also eat far less cholesterol (often less than 100 milligrams a day)[2] and less salt as well.

EATING FOR HEALTH—AND LIFE

If these numbers sound familiar, they should: They're what you get on the Pritikin Lifetime Eating Plan. When you follow our plan you get just the right amount of everything your body requires. You

FIGURE 4-1 (continued)
SOURCES OF FAT IN THE PRITIKIN PLAN
Based on less than 10% of total calories

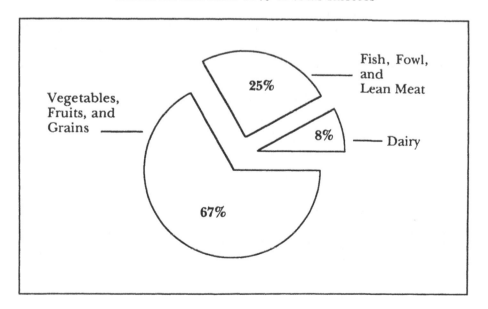

don't have to take supplements, and, as you'll soon see, you don't have to perform complicated food calculations. Where fat is concerned, staying within the 10 percent level of total calories from fat is virtually effortless: Most foods on the plan have a caloric fat content of between 5 and 15 percent, and you automatically average out to about 10 percent. Even though some of the animal protein foods on the Pritikin plan do have considerably more than 15 percent fat calories, they represent a relatively small portion of your total caloric intake. When your high-protein foods are kept to the recommended level, you'll be able to stay in the desirable overall range of 10 percent calories from fat.

This amount of dietary fat will enable you to absorb and utilize the fat-soluble vitamins from foods—namely, vitamins A, D, E, and K. While the finished form of vitamin A is found only in foods of animal origin (for example, in dairy foods), it's abundantly available as provitamin A, or beta-carotene, in yellow and orange fruits and vegetables and in leafy greens. The large quantities of beta-carotene found in plant foods are readily converted into full-fledged vitamin A in the body. In fact, a half-cup serving of carrots alone contains about 6,500 IUs (International Units) of vitamin A in the form of beta-carotene, equivalent to more than the recommended daily requirement of 2,640 to 3,300 IUs for vitamin A.

Most unrefined plant foods are also naturally good sources of vitamins E and K, and people on the lowest-fat diets throughout the world have no problems absorbing either nutrient. As for vitamin D, it's not essential that we obtain it from foods if we have exposure to sunlight all year round. But even in the absence of ultraviolet radiation, two 8-ounce glasses of vitamin D–fortified nonfat milk per day are more than enough to prevent a vitamin D deficiency in normal growing children, who need twice as much as adults do. And since the Pritikin Lifetime Eating Plan recommends two nonfat dairy servings a day (for example, two 8-ounce glasses of nonfat milk), it provides vitamin D in sufficient amounts.

FAT CATEGORIES

All fats are composed of varying amounts of saturated, monounsaturated, and polyunsaturated "fatty acids," the "building blocks" of fats. For the sake of simplicity, various sources of dietary fats are often referred to by just one of these names (for example, olive oil is known as a monounsaturated fat). In actuality, though, no naturally occurring fat has just one or two of these types of fatty acids; all are made up of a combination of the three kinds.

Fats and oils rich in monounsaturated or polyunsaturated fatty acids are liquid at room temperature, while those rich in saturated fatty acids remain solid at room temperature. Generally, the fats in most of the foods Americans typically eat are combinations of saturated and unsaturated fats, although there is usually a dominant fatty acid.

Most foods high in saturated fatty acids are animal products: Butter, whole milk, cheese, egg yolks, beef, pork, and lamb are all fairly high in saturated fatty acids, even though they contain monounsaturates and small amounts of polyunsaturates as well. Vegetable oils such as corn, safflower, sunflower, soybean, cottonseed, and sesame oils are relatively high in polyunsaturated fatty acids; olive, canola, avocado, and peanut oils, as well as most nuts, are very high in monounsaturated fatty acids.

However, there are some important exceptions to this animal/ vegetable rule, such as palm, palm-kernel, and coconut oils and cocoa butter—all very high in saturated fatty acids. Not only are these vegetable fats among the most highly saturated of all known fats, but coconut oil (the single most saturated of all) and palm oil are, unfortunately, common ingredients in many processed foods. Too often, the familiar boasts you'll find on commercial packaging— "Made with 100 percent pure vegetable shortening" and "Contains no cholesterol"—refer to foods made with either one of these highly saturated fats, which actually *raise* blood cholesterol (you'll learn more about this in Chapter 5) by provoking the liver to create *more* of it!

Fish oils, the benefits of which have been highly touted recently, consist of a blend of monounsaturated, polyunsaturated, and saturated fatty acids, although the polyunsaturated fatty acids have a chemical structure different from those in most vegetable oils.

People who follow the standard American diet get twice as much fat from saturated as from polyunsaturated sources. And while it's important to remember that all fats are harmful if eaten to excess, those foods rich in saturated fatty acids are the least desirable, because they raise serum cholesterol levels. There are no known health benefits associated with the consumption of saturated fats, but there *are* clearly established health problems associated with eating them. So of the fats you do eat, it's important that saturated fats—of both animal and vegetable origin—be kept to a minimum. And there's no easier way to do this than to follow the Pritikin plan: It contains only 2 to 3 percent saturated fatty acids, whereas the typical American diet contains 13 to 17 percent. When you compare these two ways of eating—in terms of both fat and cholesterol—the difference (and the choice!) is clear.

SATURATED FATS

While animal foods such as meat and dairy products are the most obvious sources of it, saturated fat (often disguised as hydrogenated or partially hydrogenated vegetable oil) also lurks among the ingredients in far more foods than you might suspect. As you'll see in Chapter 12 when we look closely at the labels on packaged goods, these hydrogenated or partially hydrogenated fats, as well as saturated vegetable fats such as coconut or palm oil, are some of the most pervasive ingredients in refined and processed foods. They're found in practically all breads, cakes, crackers, cookies, margarine, "health-food" and regular candy bars, presweetened breakfast cereals, egg substitutes, and nondairy creamers, to name a popular few.

Saturated fats are saturated with hydrogen. In the hydrogenation process, the double bonds of polyunsaturated or monounsaturated fats pick up more hydrogen and become more saturated. This keeps them solid and firm (or, in the case of partial hydrogenation, a bit less solid) at room temperature. This is usually done to extend the shelf life of the oils with which processed foods are made—but while the end result may be a product with a longer shelf life, it may also be a product that is more likely to shorten *your* life!

Not only do foods rich in saturated fats raise serum cholesterol levels, but they are often the very same foods (red meat and butter, for example) that contain large amounts of dietary cholesterol as well. We'll learn more about the dangers of consuming excess amounts of cholesterol in Chapter 5. For now, however, just remember that saturated fat and cholesterol often go hand in hand, and

TABLE 4-2
COMPARATIVE CSI (CHOLESTEROL/SATURATED FAT INDEX) OF DAILY INTAKES

Diet	CSI
Standard American diet	25
National Cholesterol Education Program/ American Heart Association, Step 1	18
National Cholesterol Education Program/ American Heart Association, Step 2	12
Pritikin Lifetime Eating Plan	5

As you can see, the CSI for the Pritikin Lifetime Eating Plan is significantly lower than that of the NCEP/AHA diet—it's less than half of the NCEP/AHA's *lower*-fat, *lower*-cholesterol diet! (And the CSI of the Pritikin plan is just *one-fifth* the CSI of the standard American diet.)

that it's best to minimize your intake of both saturated fatty acids *and* cholesterol. Neither is an essential nutrient and both cause or contribute to most of the major health problems in America.

In fact, almost all experts now agree that it's the *combined* content of cholesterol *and* saturated fat (sometimes expressed in terms of a Cholesterol/Saturated Fat Index, or CSI) that more accurately determines the health impact of foods (see Table 4-1).[3] Whatever the case, if you want to lower your serum cholesterol, your best move is simply to steer away from both saturated fat and cholesterol.

THE PROBLEM WITH POLYUNSATURATES

"Cholesterol-free!" polyunsaturated vegetable oils (like safflower oil) were promoted widely in the 1970s and were embraced with equal enthusiasm by millions of Americans because they lower blood levels of cholesterol. But it's important to recognize that these oils are far from a cure-all, because their cholesterol-lowering advantage is offset by known and suspected hazards.

Growing scientific evidence has linked the consumption of dietary fats, including polyunsaturated fats, to the development of obesity, a well-established risk factor for heart disease. So it certainly seems unwise to recommend diets high in polyunsaturated fats as a means of reducing cholesterol. In addition, diets high in fat of any kind (except perhaps fish oils) have been closely linked to the development of cancer—particularly breast, colon, and prostate cancer. Moreover, polyunsaturated fats are associated with gallstone formation.[4]

There has been much speculation about the chemical instability of polyunsaturated oils, which react readily with other elements, particularly oxygen, to form damaging "free radicals" and thus may render cells and tissues more susceptible to premature aging and the development of cancer. These known and suspected risks, as well as the observation that there are no human populations who have a good health record while consuming a diet high in polyunsaturated vegetable oils, are why the American Heart Association has recommended limiting the consumption of polyunsaturated oils in its overall recommendation to reduce the intake of all fats.[5]

So by all means don't be swayed by commercials that urge you to cut cholesterol by eating more margarine or vegetable oils, just because they are cholesterol-free or because of their high polyunsaturated-fat content. Both are highly processed, nutrient-poor foods that add little to your diet nutritionally.

It's important to understand that because many margarines contain partially hydrogenated vegetable oils, they actually have more saturated fat than the original oil as a result of the hydrogenation process. And, although nonhydrogenated vegetable oils don't promote cholesterol production the way saturated fats do, remember that margarines, because they *are* partially hydrogenated, may have a reduced tendency to lower cholesterol. Moreover, both margarines and oils are among the most highly refined and calorically concentrated foods you can eat: It takes almost fourteen ears of corn to produce just *one* tablespoon of corn oil! (And if you added that tablespoon of oil to a big bowl of fresh salad, brimming with vitamins, minerals, and fiber, you wouldn't add many nutrients to it—but you'd quickly double, or maybe even triple, the calories in it!)

THE OMEGA-3 MYTH

Aren't there some relatively "good"—or at least harmless—fats? Judging from recent reports, you'd think that the omega-3 fatty acids, a type of polyunsaturated fat found in cold-water seafood and in canola and soybean oils, are beneficial to your health. In fact, these fats have been so highly touted of late that some of us may be tempted to go a little too far with them. But remember that *all* fats are a highly concentrated source of calories and your body does best with very sparing amounts—amounts optimally provided by foods as they naturally exist. Fish oil (and, as you'll soon see, olive oil) is no exception: Overdosing does you no good and in fact may do you harm.

Research with such populations as the Greenland Eskimos suggests that the oils present in cold-water fish tend to lower serum triglycerides (blood fats) and discourage blood clotting. On the other hand, fish oil does not effectively lower your LDL, or "bad," cholesterol (you'll learn about "good" and "bad" cholesterol in Chapter 5); in fact, several studies have actually shown that fish-oil supplements will increase LDL cholesterol.[6,7]

If you like seafood or wish to enjoy the likely benefits of a reasonable amount of omega-3 fatty acids, substitute cold-water fish for red meat and poultry more often—but don't exceed our recommendation of $3\frac{1}{2}$ ounces of fish, lean poultry, or lean red meat a day based on the scientifically unfounded belief that "more is better." (While most "Go" foods on the Lifetime Eating Plan are virtually unlimited —unless, of course, you're following our maximal-weight-loss version —fish, meat, and dairy foods are always recommended in specific amounts.)

Fish containing the highest amounts of omega-3 include mackerel, trout, salmon, some species of tuna, halibut, and herring (in general, the colder the water, the less saturated and more polyunsaturated the fish oil will be). But eating too much of these—more than $3\frac{1}{2}$ ounces a day—puts excessive animal protein in your diet and exposes you to its many consequences, including an increased demand on the kidneys, elevated uric-acid levels, mineral loss, and possible heightened risk of thinning bones. (There is also an increasing concern about commercially caught near-shore fish, many of which have been found to be contaminated with a variety of potentially toxic or carcinogenic pollutants.[8] While the risk of eating these particular fish remains to be determined, it would obviously be related to the amount of them that you ate.)

It's important to understand that neither cold-water fish nor their omega-3 oils have any LDL-cholesterol-lowering abilities per se; in fact, their cholesterol contents are similar to those in meat. But since the ratio of fatty acids in fish is more favorable than in other sources of animal protein, making a change in your diet could help. If you normally eat meat, which contains saturated fats, substituting an equal amount of fish for the meat might cause the cholesterol output of your liver to fall slightly, and thus could lower your blood cholesterol from what it would be if you ate the meat instead of the fish. On the other hand, it's important to realize that because fish does contain both saturated fatty acids and cholesterol, the more fish you eat, the higher your serum cholesterol level will go. (In terms of cholesterol, though, as you'll learn, substituting beans for fish will lower your serum cholesterol level much more than will substituting fish for chicken or beef.)

What about fish-oil supplements? We've heard a lot about them lately, too. Not surprisingly, food sources of fish oils are best. Highly touted fish-oil supplements are calorically dense and in large amounts may also partially inhibit normal blood clotting. In addition, they may be subject to internal "rancidity reactions" that can generate within the body an excess of free radicals, the destructive molecular particles that can damage healthy cell membranes. And when given to non-insulin-dependent diabetics, fish-oil supplements have been found to raise blood sugar and increase the need for insulin.[9]

The only safe assumption we can make right now is that if you want to prevent heart disease, fish can be your first animal-protein choice—not only because of the likely omega-3 benefits, but because it has fewer saturated fatty acids than even chicken or the leanest beef. But if you have a very high cholesterol level, remember that the more fish you eat, the more you'll raise your LDL cholesterol level—whereas making beans your primary choice in the high-protein group will lower your serum cholesterol level even further than if you choose fish instead of lean poultry or lean meat.

MONOUNSATURATED FATS

Like saturated fats and cholesterol, monounsaturated fats are not dietary essentials, which means there is no nutritional need to add them to your diet. Remember that all fats are composed of varying proportions of saturated, monounsaturated, and polyunsaturated fatty acids, but various sources of dietary fats are often referred to by the name of the fatty acid that they contain in the highest percentage. Oils that contain mostly monounsaturated fats, such as olive, peanut, canola (also known as rapeseed), and avocado oils, are often promoted because they are low in saturated fats and contain no cholesterol. Their overall effect on total cholesterol is neutral. Nevertheless, recent short-term studies have shown that highly monounsaturated oils, including olive oil, reduce LDL cholesterol without reducing HDL cholesterol when they replace saturated fats.[10]

Remember, like all oils, highly monounsaturated fats such as olive oil are virtually 100 percent fat. Adding as little as two tablespoons of it to a 1,200-calorie diet that's 10 percent fat transforms that diet into one that's 25 percent fat!

DRY SKIN

One popular misconception about low-fat diets states that adding oil to your diet will help prevent dry skin. In fact, once you've met your requirements for essential fatty acids, which you will easily do on the Pritikin plan, the addition of more oil will add only to your girth. If you're concerned about dry skin, apply topical moisturizers. It's better to put the oil on the outside than on the inside!

FAKE FATS

You may have heard about some new noncaloric fat substitutes. While at first glance these "fake fats" may seem like a dream come true, there have been no conclusive studies to show that eating foods made with these substitutes instead of with real fats will help people lose weight. Moreover, the long-term effects of these fake fats have not been adequately evaluated yet.

CURRENT GUIDELINES: NEARING THE GOAL OF THE PRITIKIN PROGRAM

During the last decade, the American Heart Association and other health agencies have moved a little closer to the position of the Pritikin program on excess fat—and the trend continues. In its most recent cutback in recommended fat levels, the National Research Council affirmed that healthy American adults should limit their daily fat intake to less than 30 percent of total calories and stated that people who follow an even *lower*-fat, *lower*-cholesterol eating pattern have a "low prevalence" of heart disease.[11] Although these changes in guidelines are encouraging, we believe the best way to ensure cardiovascular health as well as to prevent obesity and breast and colon cancer is to follow the guidelines of the Pritikin program.

Now let's look at fat's companion—cholesterol—in more detail. Cholesterol is a very heated topic right now; with so many claims about doing this or that to reduce it, you're forgiven if you're confused! As with fat, you'll learn the facts—and thus how to protect yourself.

CHAPTER 5

Cholesterol: The Critical Connection

Cholesterol alert! It seems that no matter whom you talk to these days, no matter what you read or watch on television, the message is the same: Americans are *very* concerned about cholesterol.

And with good reason. Not long ago, if you had a cholesterol level of between 250 and 300 milligrams per deciliter (100 milliliters) of blood, your doctor would probably have dismissed you with a clean bill of health. But today this scenario is changing sharply. A 1986 landmark study based on more than 350,000 subjects by Dr. Jeremiah Stamler, an epidemiologist from Northwestern University, confirmed that nearly half of all fatal heart attacks among the subjects in the study resulted from cholesterol readings above 180 mg/dl.[1] For those subjects whose cholesterol levels were significantly elevated (245 mg/dl or higher), the risk of fatal heart attack was in fact at least as great as the risk from smoking and high blood pressure *combined.*

As a result of this and other new research, the National Cholesterol Education Program (NCEP) has stated that at least one in four American adults who were previously considered fit and free of risk will find out that they have a serious problem with cholesterol—and that they need to adjust their eating habits accordingly.[2] In fact, most other people who were previously considered fit and free of risk probably aren't, either: Among the people of Framingham, Massachusetts, for example, whose cardiovascular health has been

65

the subject of an ongoing study for more than forty years, only those with a cholesterol level below 150 mg/dl have been found to be free of risk for premature death due to clogged arteries.[3]

WHAT'S THE GOOD NEWS ABOUT CHOLESTEROL?

The good news is that most people, even those with seriously elevated cholesterol levels, can bring their cholesterol back down to a level that will protect them from life-threatening cardiovascular disease—without drugs. By following the Pritikin Lifetime Eating Plan, which is based on low-fat, low-cholesterol, high-unrefined-carbohydrate foods, you can keep your cholesterol level exactly where it should be for good health.

Based on our studies of thousands of individuals at the Pritikin Longevity Centers—as well as other clinical research and studies of populations where heart disease is found very infrequently—it's now clear that *for maximum cardiovascular safety, total cholesterol levels should be 100 plus your age, and no higher than 160 mg/dl.* The exception would be for individuals who have very high levels of HDLs ("good" cholesterol, which we'll learn about soon), which could push their total cholesterol level above 160 mg/dl.

Without a doubt, the surest way to keep your total serum cholesterol below 160 is to keep your intake of dietary cholesterol and saturated fat within the standards of the Pritikin plan—regardless of how many calories you consume. In fact, *most adults throughout the world who are on a lifetime eating plan that derives no more than 10 percent of its calories from fat, provides no more than 100 milligrams of cholesterol a day, and contains high-fiber, unrefined-carbohydrate foods can maintain blood cholesterol below 160 mg/dl throughout their lives.*[4]

HOW MUCH IS TOO MUCH?

The fact is that *any* cholesterol we get from food is too much; our bodies just don't need it. That's because there are actually two different methods by which serum cholesterol is elevated: through the intake of dietary cholesterol and, as we learned in Chapter 4, through the internal manufacture of cholesterol by the body itself in response to high intakes of saturated fat.

It's important to understand, first of all, that cholesterol is not an essential nutrient, which means there's no need for it in our diet. In fact, dietary cholesterol—the cholesterol found only in animal products—has been proven harmful to our arteries and has no known benefits at all. So even though cholesterol is a vital part of all of our cell membranes and is a precursor to many hormones and to vitamin D, *we don't need to eat a bit of it.* Why not? Because our cells can make all we need—even if we're on a cholesterol-free diet.

Every cell in your body is capable of making cholesterol, but by far the greatest amount is produced in the liver and intestines, which manufacture about 500 to 1,000 milligrams a day.[5] Even if you never ate any cholesterol at all, your body would still produce whatever cholesterol it needed. Remember, too, that whenever you eat foods containing saturated fat (whether they contain cholesterol or not), your liver responds by automatically overproducing cholesterol—none of which is needed—and reducing its ability to remove dietary cholesterol from the bloodstream.

It's clear that whatever cholesterol we do get from our food represents a surplus. And for most of us, sooner or later that surplus could contribute to cardiovascular disease. While most people can handle small amounts of dietary cholesterol with reasonable safety (up to about 100 milligrams a day, a little more than you'll find in $3\frac{1}{2}$ ounces of skinless chicken breast or lean beef), Americans on average consume over 400 milligrams a day—a chronic cholesterol overdose. The obvious antidote is a simple but lifesaving one: Limit our intake of animal products, since they are the only source of dietary cholesterol. But that alone isn't enough; it's essential to limit our intake of saturated fat as well. Moreover, as we'll learn shortly, to attain a truly safe serum cholesterol level we also have to increase our intake of foods that contain soluble fiber.

THE IMPACT OF EXCESS CHOLESTEROL

The problem is that the human body simply is not designed to handle excess cholesterol very well, and for some people this problem is much worse than it is for others. Population studies clearly show that when the LDL cholesterol level is over 100 (you'll learn about LDL cholesterol soon), a rise in total cholesterol level over the 160 mg/dl recommended by the Pritikin program is accompanied by an increased buildup of the atherosclerotic plaque that could eventually block the arteries.[6] And these problems are not related to age. Autopsy research has shown evidence of early development of coronary heart disease in young American soldiers killed in Korea and Vietnam: Atherosclerosis was found in over one-third of 300 soldiers autopsied in Korea,[7] and early development of atherosclerosis was found in 45 percent of 105 soldiers autopsied in Vietnam.[8] Fortunately, even though this clogging of the arteries starts early in life, it's a disease that develops slowly. Unfortunately, however, atherosclerosis displays no symptoms as it gradually restricts blood flow—until it reaches the life-threatening point (see Figure 5-1). In fact, consider that cardiovascular disease claims well over half a million lives each year.

The most recent (1988) cholesterol guidelines announced by the National Cholesterol Education Program state that a "desirable" total serum cholesterol is one that falls *below* 200 mg/dl, a "borderline high" is from 200 to 239, and any cholesterol reading over 240 mg/dl is "unacceptably high" and in need of treatment.[9] This is a far cry from the 250 to 300 that used to be considered acceptable. Nevertheless, thousands of people with serum cholesterol levels between 160 and 200 mg/dl still die from cardiovascular disease every year, which is why we feel strongly that the Pritikin program's guideline for a desirable cholesterol level—less than 160 mg/dl—is what is needed in order to save more lives. But the fact is that most people cannot attain this truly safe serum cholesterol level by following the relatively liberal NCEP/AHA dietary guidelines, and as a result many

FIGURE 5-1
THE NATURAL HISTORY OF ATHEROSCLEROSIS

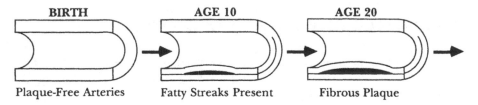

BIRTH	AGE 10	AGE 20
Plaque-Free Arteries	Fatty Streaks Present	Fibrous Plaque

people will have to take expensive and potentially harmful cholesterol-lowering drugs in an attempt to do so. We offer a healthy alternative.

THE HEALTHY SOLUTION

Over thirty years ago, Nathan Pritikin was already convinced that the link to heart disease was a dietary one. Based on his own careful studies of the diets, medical histories, and death rates of a variety of populations, he concluded that excess dietary fat, cholesterol, and salt were behind the astonishing incidence of high serum cholesterol, coronary heart disease, and high blood pressure in many cultures. By contrast, he realized, low intakes of fat, cholesterol, and salt were associated with a very low incidence of cardiovascular problems.

Time and solid scientific research have only confirmed his conclusions. The beneficial effect of lowered total and LDL cholesterol levels on coronary health has been demonstrated clearly by Dr. David Blankenhorn at the University of Southern California, who showed that by marked reduction of blood cholesterol, coronary heart disease could be slowed, stopped, or even made to regress,[10] and by the National Heart, Lung and Blood Institute's Lipid Research Clinic, which clearly demonstrated that every 1 percent drop in serum cholesterol led to a 2 percent decrease in the risk of heart disease.[11] In perhaps the most famous long-term cholesterol study of all, conducted over a forty-year period in Framingham, Massachusetts, Dr. William Castelli has shown that the risk of heart attack begins to rise gradually at a total cholesterol level of 150, then increases more steeply as cholesterol exceeds 200.[12] But, Dr. Castelli

FIGURE 5-1 (continued)

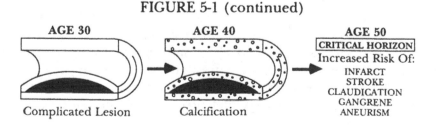

AGE 30 — Complicated Lesion

AGE 40 — Calcification

AGE 50 — CRITICAL HORIZON — Increased Risk Of: INFARCT, STROKE, CLAUDICATION, GANGRENE, ANEURISM

reports, during all the years of the Framingham study they have yet to see a heart attack in anyone with a cholesterol level below 150![13]

The link between low cholesterol and coronary health has been taken even further in the work of Dr. Dean Ornish at the University of California School of Medicine in San Francisco. Dr. Ornish has demonstrated that without the use of cholesterol-lowering drugs, a program like the Pritikin program, consisting of a low-fat, low-sodium, low-cholesterol, and high-fiber eating plan, moderate exercise, life-style management, and cessation of smoking, not only can halt but can actually *reverse* the atherosclerotic effects of coronary heart disease.[14]

It's now overwhelmingly clear that one of the major risk factors for coronary heart disease is elevated blood cholesterol. Controlling your dietary cholesterol and saturated-fat intake is the most effective way to reduce this risk, but other factors—smoking, hypertension, diabetes, and not excerising regularly—can pose major threats to your health as well. While people who have safe levels of serum cholesterol are clearly in far less danger—even if they smoke, pay no attention to the signs of high blood pressure, and forgo exercise for a sedentary life-style—it is critical to acknowledge that smoking, high blood pressure, and a sedentary life-style are still dangerous and can greatly increase your chances of dying from a stroke, cancer, or other serious disease.

HOW FOOD AFFECTS YOUR CHOLESTEROL LEVEL

Saturated fat in all its forms is the single most potent dietary influence on total and LDL cholesterol levels. Whether it's found in animal foods (as in meats and dairy products) or vegetable sources (as in coconut oil, palm oil, cocoa butter, and hydrogenated vegetable oils), consuming an excess of foods high in saturated fat can have disastrous effects on your serum cholesterol level.

Why? First of all, most foods high in saturated fat also contain cholesterol. But even if they don't, saturated fats cause your liver to produce excessive cholesterol, which you don't need. In addition, too much fat of any kind in your diet promotes obesity and excess body fat—which, in turn, raises your cholesterol level even higher. On average, each 10-pound weight gain is associated with an increase in serum cholesterol of approximately 5 mg/dl.

Some of what you eat won't make much difference one way or the other (although that's not a license to overdo it!). Refined starchy foods (like cornstarch, potato starch, and white rice), from which most or all of the cholesterol-lowering fiber has been removed, won't raise cholesterol, but they won't help to lower it either. The same is true for refined sugars. And despite recent claims, refined oils high in monounsaturated fats, like olive oil, won't help to lower your serum cholesterol level either, unless they replace foods that are high in saturated fats and/or cholesterol. What's more, refined oils and refined carbohydrates are nutritionally empty: They'll add needless calories to your diet, but few, if any, essential nutrients.

FOODS THAT AFFECT YOUR CHOLESTEROL LEVEL

Decrease Cholesterol

Recommended foods that may help decrease blood cholesterol include fruit, vegetables, beans, peas, oats, barley, and sweet potatoes. Although a food or food component may decrease cholesterol, it may not be recommended on the Pritikin Lifetime Eating Plan for other reasons. For example, diets high in polyunsaturated fats may lower cholesterol; however, high-fat diets are associated with obesity and a greater risk of certain cancers.

Increase Cholesterol

Some foods that can dramatically increase your cholesterol level if consumed in sufficient amounts include tropical oils, egg yolks, butter, lard, hydrogenated fats, and shortening. Even foods that are acceptable on the Pritikin Lifetime Eating Plan—such as fish, poultry, or lean meat—have the potential to increase your blood cholesterol level. To keep your blood cholesterol at a reasonably safe level, the recommended portions of these foods and nonfat dairy products is controlled. Remember you can eat too much of a good thing.

Little or No Effect
Foods that have little or no effect on blood cholesterol levels include monounsaturated fats, refined sugars, refined starches, and alcohol.

HOW FOODS DECREASE CHOLESTEROL

When it comes to curbing cholesterol, choosing to limit or avoid certain foods is not the whole story: Adding certain beneficial items to your eating plan can actively keep blood levels under control. Recent studies have found that beans, peas, lentils, oats, yams, barley, and most vegetables and fruits contain soluble fibers that have been shown to actively lower serum cholesterol. The gums and pectins found in these foods may increase the excretion of cholesterol-derived bile acids, and thereby promote the net excretion of cholesterol from the body. Just like certain cholesterol-lowering drugs (but without the danger of harmful side effects!), the fibers found in these foods allow more cholesterol to be converted to bile acids, which can then be excreted from the body. Here's how: Soluble fiber binds with bile acids, depleting the liver's supply of them and causing it to produce more, using its own cholesterol. When the liver's supply of cholesterol is depleted, it extracts LDL cholesterol from the bloodstream to build up its store of cholesterol again. And soluble fibers also delay the absorption of carbohydrates and thereby lower serum insulin levels, which research suggests may help reduce cholesterol synthesis by the liver.

CHOLESTEROL FRACTIONS

Perhaps you recently had a cholesterol test, and when you got the results you were given three different numbers: total cholesterol, HDL cholesterol (high-density lipoprotein, often referred to as "good" cholesterol), and LDL cholesterol (low-density lipoprotein, often referred to as "bad" cholesterol). It's not hard to understand these readings. In terms of milligrams of cholesterol per deciliter (100 milliliters) of blood, total cholesterol is made up of HDLs,

LDLs, and other cholesterol "fractions," although the greatest portion is represented by LDLs and HDLs.

You've probably heard that it's important to have high levels of "good" HDL cholesterol in your system, along with the lowest possible amount of "bad" LDL cholesterol. What's the difference between these two kinds of cholesterol, anyway? What about cholesterol "ratios"? And why is total cholesterol important?

CHOLESTEROL: THE GOOD AND THE BAD

Let's take a closer look at these cholesterol "fractions," and at what makes HDLs "good" and LDLs "bad." After you have fasted, a blood test will show three carriers of cholesterol: HDLs, LDLs, and very-low-density lipoproteins, or VLDLs. LDL cholesterol usually makes up about 65 percent of total cholesterol; about 20 percent circulates as HDL, and the remainder of total cholesterol is VLDL.

Cholesterol is a white, waxy substance that cannot dissolve in water; neither can it dissolve in blood, which is mostly water. But cholesterol has to get to the cells where it may be needed, so a fleet of special water-soluble carriers called lipoproteins—literally, molecules of fat linked with protein—are used to transport cholesterol and other water-insoluble products (like triglycerides, which are blood fats) throughout the bloodstream. Thus, although HDL and LDL are sometimes respectively thought of as "good" and "bad" cholesterol, they are, more precisely, cholesterol *carriers*. In fact, the actual cholesterol molecules found in HDL, LDL, and VLDL are really the same. What's crucial to our understanding of how cholesterol is metabolized is *how* these lipoproteins do their carrying.

First, very-low-density lipoproteins are secreted by the liver into the bloodstream, where they carry triglycerides (which come from the diet or are produced by the liver), primarily to the fat cells. They also carry cholesterol produced in the liver or coming from the diet. The VLDLs actually contain five times more triglycerides than cholesterol, but as they travel through the bloodstream they are broken down by enzymes which release the triglycerides. As the triglyceride is removed from the VLDL particle, the particle becomes concentrated with cholesterol. Eventually some of this VLDL particle is converted to low-density ("bad") lipoprotein, which delivers cholesterol directly to cells. If the serum level of LDL cholesterol is elevated, some of it will end up in the cells of the arterial walls, where it triggers the growth of atherosclerotic plaque (see Figure 5-1 on pages 68–69). And if LDL cholesterol remains high for many years, this plaque eventually blocks blood flow and can trigger a heart attack or stroke.

By contrast, HDLs, or "good" cholesterol, appear to act as scavengers that seek out excess cellular cholesterol and usher it away from tissues and arteries and back to the liver, where it enters the liver's cholesterol pool and can be used for bile acids.

So, while HDLs appear to play a beneficial role in partially counteracting the harmful effects of too much LDL, the public is receiving a distorted message about these "good" high-density lipoproteins. The facts are that HDL levels are determined primarily by genetic factors; that the only safe ways to increase them are to quit smoking, lose weight, and exercise; and that high-fat diets are associated with increased levels of both HDL and total cholesterol, resulting in more deaths from atherosclerosis.[15] *What's best is to have low total cholesterol and the lowest possible level of LDLs as well.* Once you achieve this, you won't have to worry about not having enough "good" cholesterol, because when your total cholesterol is 160 mg/dl or less, and/or your LDLs are below 100 mg/dl, a somewhat lower HDL figure loses most of its risk significance. In this "cholesterol safety zone," minimal risk is associated with lower than average HDLs. This stands to reason, because if you don't have excess cholesterol in your bloodstream and tissues, you don't have as much need for the scavenging efforts of HDLs.

THE TARAHUMARAS: A CASE IN POINT

This point is demonstrated by the remarkable coronary health of the Tarahumara Indians of Mexico. The average American HDL level is 45 for men and 55 for women, and values much below 35 are considered an increased risk for coronary heart disease. But the Tarahumaras have HDL levels averaging "only" between 22 and 32 mg/dl. However, their *total* cholesterol levels are only between 120 and 150.[16] The Tarahumaras' HDL averages would be considered dangerously low by many Western clinicians if compared, for example, with the average American HDL range of 45 to 55—but because the Tarahumaras' LDL cholesterol levels are below 100 mg/dl, and most have a total cholesterol level below 150, they are at minimal risk for heart attacks or strokes.

And, of course, it's important to remember that under certain circumstances high HDL levels are no guarantee of good health: To look at another population, men in east Finland have high HDL levels—and also very high death rates from coronary heart disease.[17] Because their total cholesterol levels are so high, their high HDLs simply aren't taking care of the problem.

CHOLESTEROL RATIOS

Often when cholesterol tests are performed laboratories will indicate, in addition to total, HDL, and LDL cholesterol readings, the ratio of total cholesterol to HDL cholesterol. Although nearly all experts now agree that it's far more important to look at total cholesterol and LDL levels than at this ratio, there's still so much talk of ratios that it's helpful to understand what they mean. Also, if your total cholesterol is over 160 mg/dl, the ratio is a useful way to assess your risk for coronary heart disease.

The average American ratio of total to HDL cholesterol is about 5 to 1. For any given serum cholesterol, ratios below 5 are associated with a lower risk of coronary heart disease and ratios above 5 with an increased risk. But what if your total cholesterol level were 150 and your HDL cholesterol level only 25? This would give you a total-to-HDL ratio of 6, yet your risk of heart attack would be extremely low because your total cholesterol level and your LDL cholesterol level are so low.

On the other hand, though, if your total cholesterol were 300 mg/dl and your HDL were 75, your ratio would be 4—and if you were to look only at the ratio, your risk of cardiovascular disease might appear to be lower. But in fact your risk of having a heart attack would be much higher than average—even though your HDL and the ratio looked okay—because your total cholesterol and LDL cholesterol are too high. Of course, if someone with the same 300 mg/dl total cholesterol had an HDL of 25 instead of 75, the risk of a heart attack would be much higher still. Once you realize that diet has more of an impact on LDL and total cholesterol than it does on HDL, you'll realize that focusing on HDL and the ratio of total cholesterol to HDL cholesterol can be very misleading.

It's important to understand, too, that whatever the ratio, it can give the wrong impression when HDL levels are low but total cholesterol and LDL are also low. To use the Tarahumaras as an example again, among these Indians the ratio of total cholesterol to HDL is typically 5, the same as the typical American ratio; yet the risk of coronary heart disease among these people is vastly lower than among Americans because the Tarahumaras' *total* and LDL cholesterol levels are so low.

Keep in mind that a low-fat, low-cholesterol, high-fiber diet will maximally reduce your total cholesterol. Most of this reduction will be of the LDLs, but your HDLs may also drop. However, you shouldn't be concerned over a drop in your "good" cholesterol level under these circumstances, because your ratio of total cholesterol to HDL will also tend to improve. A low HDL level only becomes more significant when your LDLs exceed 100 mg/dl, or when your ratio of total cholesterol to HDL is not improving. At that point you may want to consult your doctor, because you may still be at some risk for cardiovascular disease.

But rather than worry about a drop in HDL or an unfavorable ratio, it's far better to focus instead on something you have more control over, such as lowering your total and your LDL levels—then you won't have *anything* to worry about.

WHEN HIGH HDL'S HELP

For people on a high-fat, high-cholesterol diet, elevated HDLs do correspond to a reduced risk for heart disease. Those who have more HDL "escorts" at their disposal will be at an obvious advantage over their low-HDL counterparts with the same total cholesterol.

How high should HDLs be for those on a high-fat, high-cholesterol diet? Most experts agree that when both total and LDL cholesterol levels are too high, an HDL level below 35 mg/dl represents an additional risk factor for coronary heart disease.[18] For example, a total cholesterol of 250 and an HDL of 55 (for a ratio of 4.5) is clearly preferable to a total cholesterol of 250 and an HDL of only 25 (which gives a ratio of 10).

CAN YOU CHANGE YOUR CHOLESTEROL FRACTIONS?

As a practical matter, on the Pritikin program we emphasize the greater importance of lowering LDL cholesterol over raising HDL cholesterol, because as it turns out there's little you can do to appreciably raise your HDL cholesterol. Certainly cessation of smoking, weight reduction, and aerobic exercise can modestly increase HDL values, but beyond that you'd have to resort to certain medications to increase your HDL more substantially. Obviously, until this approach can be tested far more thoroughly it remains a potentially risky one. It might appear that an easy way to raise your HDL cholesterol level is to switch to a diet high in monounsaturated fats. But this won't really help you, because high-*fat* diets can have other negative consequences of their own, including obesity and an increased risk of breast and colon cancer. On the other hand, we do know precisely how to reduce both total and LDL values and improve ratios to bring them to optimal levels: by incorporating the principles of the Pritikin Lifetime Eating Plan.

THE SAFEST ALTERNATIVE

The very best way to keep total blood cholesterol and LDL cholesterol levels down is by directly curtailing your intake of saturated fats and dietary cholesterol while simultaneously increasing your intake of minimally processed carbohydrates that are rich in soluble fiber, which, as we'll learn soon, also help to suppress cholesterol absorption and/or synthesis.

Taking cholesterol-lowering drugs while you're on the standard American diet is definitely *not* the safest solution! Besides risking adverse side effects, relying on medications will do nothing to change the poor food choices that led to high serum cholesterol in the first place. What's worse, sticking to a diet that raises your cholesterol level (in the mistaken belief that you can undo all the cholesterol damage with medication) also increases your risk for the development of obesity, hypertension, adult-onset diabetes, and certain types of cancer. And the drugs will do nothing to alter your risk factors for *these* diseases!

Moreover, research tells us that even when dietary cholesterol does not increase serum cholesterol there's a possibility that it may promote atherosclerosis. Exactly how dietary cholesterol can be atherogenic independent of its effect on serum cholesterol levels is still a matter of debate, but four recent studies all showed a much greater increase in cardiovascular-disease deaths in people who consumed a high level of dietary cholesterol.[19]

A HIDDEN THREAT

What if you're one of those "lucky" people who seems to be able to eat everything from eggs Benedict to ice cream and still maintain a surprisingly low blood cholesterol level? Well, you may not be as lucky as you think. As we just learned, research shows you could still be headed for (or may already have) quite a bit of atherosclerosis anyway. Here's the prevailing thought on why.

After you've eaten a meal that's high in fat, your body produces lipoprotein carriers called chylomicrons to aid in the transport of the ingested fats and cholesterol through your bloodstream. These carriers, like low-density-lipoprotein (LDL, or "bad," cholesterol) carriers, are thought to become highly atherogenic: According to theory, once they are partially broken down and become enriched with dietary cholesterol, chylomicron remnants are able to deposit their cholesterol directly onto your arterial walls.[20] But because chylomicrons appear only for eight to ten hours after a high-fat meal, they do *not* show up on a fasting cholesterol test. Even if serum cholesterol is measured four to six hours after a high-fat meal (when these chylomicron remnants are present), it will be increased only slightly.

So how do you avoid the hidden threat of dietary cholesterol? The obvious answer, of course, is to watch what you eat! Remember that *all* the cholesterol you eat is excess, so if you don't limit your daily cholesterol intake, anything containing cholesterol—even low-fat poultry or fish—can threaten your arteries, because eating excess cholesterol is significantly related to long-term risk of coronary heart disease—no matter what your serum cholesterol level may be.[21] For most people, consuming no more than 100 milligrams of dietary cholesterol a day (roughly the amount found in $3\frac{1}{2}$ ounces of fish, lean poultry, or lean meat) is reasonably safe. And that is exactly our "prescription."

EATING NO CHOLESTEROL

What would happen if you ate *no* cholesterol at all? Since you have no need for any outside source, your liver and other tissues would simply produce what they needed anyway. However, unless you're a *strict* vegetarian you might want to include some animal foods (including nonfat dairy foods) in your meals, because they're an important source of vitamins D and B_{12}, which are not found in vegetable foods. Also, many of us have developed a taste for such foods, and they add flavor and palatability to our dishes. (If you're a strict vegetarian, alternate sources of B_{12} include supplements and some fortified breakfast cereals; vitamin D you can get from the sun.)

It's not hard to ensure that you're consuming fairly safe levels of cholesterol—just follow the Pritikin Lifetime Eating Plan. And if your serum cholesterol level is too high, you've got the best possible chance of lowering it through diet alone simply by enjoying the delicious and versatile menus we offer. Our studies have shown that after three weeks at a Pritikin Longevity Center, the average participant experiences a drop in serum cholesterol of 25 percent.[22,23] Those who had a beginning cholesterol level in excess of 265 mg/dl had an average drop of 31 percent.[24] This means that on the average, people cut their risk of heart disease by 50 percent; those with a beginning cholesterol level over 265 mg/dl cut their risk by 60 percent or more![25] Most people whose cholesterol levels are too high and who then adopt the Pritikin program will find a much bigger drop in total cholesterol and LDL cholesterol than they could ever hope to achieve with the National Cholesterol Education Program/American Heart Association diet.

WHAT'S MOST IMPORTANT

There's so much information available nowadays on cholesterol—some of it helpful, some of it confusing, some of it actually misleading. To make things easier, just concentrate on these most important cholesterol facts:

- Your total blood cholesterol and LDL cholesterol are the most telling measures of your risk for heart disease. The best way to lower both levels is to reduce the amount of saturated fat and cholesterol you eat every day and to increase your consumption of foods rich in soluble fiber.
- A small minority of people are unable to achieve a safe cholesterol level without the use of drugs. Though effective, all cholesterol-lowering drugs have side effects and should be used only after giving a low-fat, low-cholesterol, high-fiber diet a fair trial. And remember, if you *are* taking cholesterol-lowering drugs, the better your diet, the lower the dosage—and the lower the risk of side effects.
- For maximum protection from heart and blood-vessel disease, your total cholesterol should not exceed 100 plus your age, and should never be higher than 160 mg/dl (unless your HDL is so high it pushes your total up).
- Just because your HDL figure is high, this doesn't mean you're safe if your LDL cholesterol is also high. A high HDL cholesterol level will reduce but will not neutralize the risk of heart disease associated with a simultaneously elevated LDL cholesterol level.
- While your best defense is to lower your total cholesterol and LDL cholesterol, it is known that you can safely raise your HDL cholesterol somewhat by reducing body fat, giving up smoking, and doing regular aerobic exercise.
- While they are lower in saturated fat, lean poultry and fish do not contain much less cholesterol than do lean meats, so it's best to eat no more than $3\frac{1}{2}$ ounces of any of these foods a day. In the high-protein category, fish is recommended over poultry since studies show a reduced risk of coronary heart disease in individuals consuming a modest amount of fish per week instead of meat, compared to those consuming meat only, and no fish at all, as their high-protein food.[26]

• Include more soluble fiber in your meals—especially oats, barley, legumes, yams, sweet potatoes, fruits, and vegetables—to help lower your serum cholesterol.

Now you've got the facts—in easily digestible form! Next on our fact-finding tour is an exploration of something that you may be consuming far more of than you realize and far more of than you need: salt.

CHAPTER 6

Shaking Out the Salt

Do you know what your food is *really* supposed to taste like?

Well, even if you think you do, you're in for a pleasant surprise. Because after only a month or two on the healthful Pritikin Lifetime Eating Plan, you'll soon discover another delightful dividend: Your taste buds will start to come alive!

You may have long since forgotten what food tastes like when it hasn't been doused with sugar or salt. But it wouldn't be your fault: For decades, commercially prepared processed foods haven't given you much choice. As you'll see when we learn about label reading, it's sometimes hard to find a brand-name food whose list of ingredients *doesn't* include an "-ose" (meaning sugar) or a "sodium" (usually sodium chloride, which is common table salt). In fact, no alleged "taste enhancer" is added to foods more frequently than salt.

Before we go on, though, let's clarify these two important terms, *sodium* and *salt*. Though often used interchangeably in everyday conversation, these aren't actually the same. One, however, is a component of the other: Sodium accounts for about 40 percent of sodium chloride, which we know as table salt.

If you're like most Americans, you've probably been consuming far more salt than your body needs without ever being aware of it. For one thing, reaching for the saltshaker may be so routine by now that you just sprinkle away before you've even tasted what's on your plate. Then, of course, there's the problem with "convenience" foods: Far too much salt—as well as other sodium compounds, such

82

as monosodium glutamate (MSG), baking soda, or sodium nitrate—may already have been added to these items, even if you don't add any more yourself.

Does it matter? If it tastes fine the way it comes out of the can, should you be concerned? As you've seen with every other nutrient we've covered, there's a good and a bad side to nearly everything we eat. We *need* small amounts of essential fats, and you'll see that protein is necessary in modest amounts. The problem is that we consume too *much* of what we need, and so it is with salt: The human body does need a small amount of sodium, but when it gets too much of it in the form of salt—sodium chloride—serious problems can ensue.

But before we get to the serious health risks that excess dietary salt can create, let's savor the good news just a little longer: Fresh, minimally processed, healthy food actually has *more* taste—more specific, natural taste—than oversalted or highly processed food. That's because the real flavor of each different food comes through. Let's face it: All oversalted food tastes the same—salty! But fresh foods that aren't masked with a lot of sodium-based "flavor enhancers," such as salt or MSG, have a distinct, wonderful taste of their own—which will come as a delightful surprise to anyone who's never eaten this way before.

As you've already begun to discover if you've been following the Lifetime Eating Plan, foods like corn on the cob *without* salt and butter are an entirely new experience: They're deliciously naturally sweet. Vegetables like broccoli, squash, spinach, and carrots all have subtle flavors you may never have fully enjoyed—until you put down the salt. And the lovely nuttiness of whole-grain bread and pasta doesn't need any "enhancing" at all, least of all with salt, which only masks the natural sweetness of these healthy foods. (In fact, the highly corrosive properties of salt can damage your taste buds as well, making it all the more difficult to really taste what you're eating. Removing the excess salt from your diet will help change all that.)

When you do want to add some "zip" to foods, though, you've got any number of options apart from salt. Healthy cuisine is definitely not drab! Spices, herbs, and condiments are exciting elements of cooking according to the Pritikin plan, and are yours to use with as much imagination as you've got. But if you've relied on salt or other sodium-based seasonings for a long time, you might want to start out by tasting the unadorned foods themselves, undoctored by anything—perhaps for the first time in your life. Very soon, you'll see how unnecessary all those automatic pinches of salt were!

SODIUM BASICS

Sodium is actually a nutrient vital to the saline solution that makes up our body's fluids. Like chloride and potassium, sodium is an electrolyte critical to the electrical activity of our body's cells, especially our nerve and heart-muscle cells. These electrolytes are also needed for a variety of metabolic functions. But an excess of salt (which, by the way, accounts for 90 percent of the sodium in the typical American diet) has been associated with high blood pressure, stomach cancer, and strokes.[1]

The human body actually needs only about 250 to 500 milligrams of dietary sodium a day—no more sodium than you'd find in one-fifth of a *teaspoon* of salt, and an amount that's easily provided by the unprocessed foods emphasized on the Pritikin plan (without adding any salt at all). Yet the average dose of sodium in this country is anywhere from 4,000 to 6,000 milligrams a day—twenty times the required amount!

Now *that* is an excess. But why is it so dangerous? To begin with, too much salt can contribute to or aggravate health problems such as stomach cancer, angina, and congestive heart failure. It may also increase calcium excretion and thus may heighten the risk of osteoporosis.[2] But the *big* risk is hypertension—high blood pressure.

As far back as the early 1900s, scientists suspected a link between a high intake of sodium chloride (and perhaps other sodium-based compounds) and high blood pressure. So you've undoubtedly heard of the connection between sodium and hypertension, and if you suffer from high blood pressure you've probably already been told to cut down your salt intake. But even if you don't currently suffer from hypertension, read on: You'll soon see that you may not be as immune as you thought to the ultimate dangers of excess salt.

SALT AND HIGH BLOOD PRESSURE

The flow of blood created by the rhythmic pumping of your heart exerts a natural pressure on your artery walls; this is what's known as blood pressure. If your blood volume is within a normal range, and if the tension within the muscle surrounding the artery wall is normal, your pressure should likewise be safe (in fact, pressure that's extremely low can be very serious or even life-threatening). But if your blood volume is increased beyond a safe level, as can happen if you consume too much salt, hypertension develops: The additional blood volume puts extra pressure on your arteries, and your blood pressure rises, possibly to a dangerous level.

There are actually two types of high blood pressure: primary (or essential) hypertension, and secondary hypertension. The exact cause of the first is not known, but excessive salt—or possibly sodium—intake may be an important factor. Secondary hypertension, on the other hand, has its origins in an underlying disorder such as kidney disease or hyperthyroidism.

In the vast majority of cases, hypertension is "primary," and appears to be influenced largely by eating and life-style habits—especially by a diet high in salt as well as in fat (although obesity, alcohol consumption, and a sedentary life-style may also contribute to increased blood pressure).

Other factors have an effect on blood pressure, too: Emotional or physical stress will make your blood pressure rise temporarily; in fact, it's a normal reaction. However, if the source of the stress goes away and your blood pressure *remains* high, then you've got a problem. For people who fall into this group, salt may be a primary villain.

How exactly can too much salt contribute to high blood pressure? While our kidneys are designed to dispose of excess sodium, when we overwork these natural filters with enormous amounts of sodium in the form of salt, they may become less efficient at their cleanup job over time. And because our bodies seek to maintain an unchanged concentration of sodium, if excess sodium is not excreted it will prompt the fluid retention necessary to keep this sodium concentration in balance. Blood volume then increases as one result of this additional fluid.

SALT AND OTHER POPULATIONS

Without exception, studies of populations where salt consumption is low show little or no evidence of essential hypertension or its related ills—heart and kidney disease and stroke. But salty foods do not usually act alone. In fact, hypertension is a problem only in regions where salty foods and/or foods high in saturated fat are standard fare: Saturated fat actually appears to augment the blood-pressure-raising effects of excessive salt.[3]

In fact, the Japanese provide two good examples of the effects diet can have on all-around health: On a traditional diet low in fat but unusually high in salt (a major component of soy sauce, a staple of the Japanese diet), the Japanese have long shown a higher incidence of hypertension than do people who consume more fat and less salt. In response to this serious concern, recent public health measures to reduce salt use and increase blood-pressure medication in Japan have resulted in a significant decline in hypertension and stroke. Ironically, however, the simultaneous Westernization of Japanese cuisine has resulted in increased consumption of fat and cholesterol, and with them, an increase in serum cholesterol among today's Japanese.

WHAT'S THE REAL CULPRIT?

Is it salt or sodium? Does it make a difference? Let's take a closer look. We do know that too much *salt*—sodium chloride—elevates blood pressure, but scientists have debated whether this is triggered by too much *sodium* itself or by sodium *in combination with chloride* in table salt. (For example, some preliminary research suggests that sodium salts other than sodium chloride are much less likely to cause hypertension, but the evidence is not yet conclusive.[4]) Whatever the case, since most of the sodium in the standard American diet is chemically combined with chloride in the form of salt anyway, the clear indication is that we should steer clear of excessive salt.

But we can't stop with salt, because, as we've said, saturated fat is also a factor. So is it salt, or is it *fat*—or both? We know that a diet rich in fats and high in salt is the one most apt to increase blood pressure to possibly dangerous levels.[5] So it's not surprising, then, that removing saturated and total fat from the diet seems to be what causes the dramatic blood-pressure drop in people who follow the Lifetime Eating Plan, which is low in salt and all types of fat, but especially saturated fat. At the Pritikin Longevity Centers, we've found that when put on a low-salt, low-fat diet, 83 percent of hypertensives were able to discontinue their medication, yet maintain normal blood pressure.[6]

Naturally, this doesn't mean you should add salt to your food if you're not salt sensitive, because continued use of salt may cause your blood pressure to go higher *with time,* and excess salt can do other damage besides raising blood pressure. It simply shows, once again, that hypertension has more than one variable.

If your blood pressure is too high, you can probably bring it down to a safe level, keep it under control, and possibly discontinue your medication as well by following the Pritikin program. On the other hand, if your blood pressure is normal now, you can make sure it stays that way by following the Lifetime Eating Plan, exercising regularly (with your doctor's approval, of course), and managing stress as successfully as possible. And since there's no foolproof way to predict who will be able to tolerate a lifetime of high-salt eating without ill effects, cutting back on salt makes sense for *everyone.*

COUNTERACTING SODIUM WITH POTASSIUM

Because potassium tends to promote the excretion of sodium from the body—thereby decreasing the amount of fluid needed between cells and reducing blood volume—it may counteract to some extent the hypertensive effects of excess salt. And, not surprisingly, there is some epidemiological evidence to suggest that a potassium-deficient diet may aggravate the blood-pressure-raising effects of excessive salt.[7]

For example, one study found that vegetarians had markedly lower blood pressures than did a control group on a typical Western diet, even though both consumed similar amounts of sodium.[8] The vegetarians (who also ate far less fat as well as more carbohydrates) had a potassium intake nearly double that of the control group. (Refined grain products, sugar, refined fats, oils, and alcoholic beverages—which are often abundant on the typical American diet—are all low-potassium foods, and several of these refined products are also notoriously high in sodium.)

Because the Pritikin plan is already low in sodium—*and* provides an adequate supply of potassium, is low in fat and alcohol, facilitates maintenance of an ideal body weight, and provides a beneficial ratio of polyunsaturated to saturated fat—it works well all around. It also mirrors the diet that the earliest humans evolved on, which seems to have consisted largely of tubers, beans, vegetables, and fruits, all of which are naturally low in sodium and high in potassium; even when meat was consumed, it is not likely that sodium intake exceeded 700 milligrams a day.[9]

MAKING YOUR LOW-SALT DIET PERMANENT

Now that you know the benefits of a low-salt diet, and the dangers of a high-salt one, you probably don't need a lot of encouragement to limit your salt intake. Wherever you eat—at home, in a restaurant, or on the road on business—keep the following tips for low-sodium eating in mind:

- Limit your intake to a daily average of approximately 1 milligram of sodium per calorie, up to a maximum of 1,600 milligrams a day. For example, if you were consuming about 1,600 calories a day, that would amount to approximately 1,600 milligrams of sodium. This is simple to do on the Pritikin Lifetime Eating Plan, where many of the fruits and vegetables you eat contain much less than 1 milligram of sodium per calorie.
- Minimize your intake of highly refined and processed foods, which are usually not only high in sodium but also low in potassium (as well as in magnesium and calcium, which, with potassium, may also be essential for regulating blood pressure).
- Potassium is found in all fruits and vegetables, although bananas, apples, oranges, honeydew, cantaloupe, apricots, and mushrooms contain the most.
- When choosing "convenience" foods—whether canned, frozen, bot-

tled, or boxed—avoid highly salted, smoked, and pickled items, which are high in sodium, and shop for low-sodium alternatives.
- Any items that offer ingredient and nutrition information are now required by the federal government to spell out the sodium content in milligrams per serving. Also, all food products that make a controlled-sodium claim must conform to the following Food and Drug Administration standards for labeling:

"Sodium-free" means the product contains less than 5 milligrams of sodium per serving.
"Very Low Sodium" means no more than 35 milligrams per serving.
"Low Sodium" has no more than 140 milligrams of sodium per serving.
"Reduced Sodium" has 75 percent less sodium than its regular counterpart.
"No Salt Added" means that no extra salt has been added for flavor, but it still may have been processed with salt or sodium compounds.

These claims, particularly "No Salt Added," can be very misleading, so be sure to read the entire label to avoid being confused.
- Watch your intake not only of table salt (sodium chloride), but also of sea salt; kelp; baking soda; baking powder; onion, garlic, and celery salt; monosodium glutamate (MSG); sodium saccharin, sodium nitrate, sodium propionate, and any other ingredient with "sodium" in its name. The same "watch" applies to ketchup, chili sauce, barbecue sauce, Worcestershire sauce, capers, cooking wines, and miso. Even sodium-reduced soy sauce and tamari are highly salted, as are most prepared mustards, so we suggest using no more than a teaspoon of such seasonings a day.
- If you are in training for sports or do any heavy exercise, do *not* add more salt to your meals, and do not take salt tablets.

MAKE FOOD TASTE GREAT WITHOUT SALT!

Of course, the most pleasant part of low-sodium eating is the fact that it's delicious! Not only will your taste buds adjust to the absence of all that salt, but they'll absolutely revel in the world of new flavors. Thanks to the availability of a growing number of less salty convenience foods (foods that simply weren't on the shelves as recently as three or four years ago), it's easier than ever to enjoy good low-sodium eating. You'll find low-sodium versions of baking powder, bread crumbs, ketchup, mustard, tomato sauce, tomato paste, canned and frozen vegetables, canned fish (such as tuna and salmon), canned soups and beans, breads, crackers, and cereals—just keep your eyes open! Haunt your neighborhood health-food store as well as your supermarket.

In Chapter 12 you'll find a comprehensive herb and spice chart to give you new ideas about exciting seasonings. But get your mind going now: Think of how interesting tonight's broiled chicken would be with chopped cilantro, fresh onion, and salsa instead of salt. Or plan now to season your next piece of poached fish with chopped dill, fresh lemon, and a bit of dry mustard. Other enticing alternatives to salt include freshly ground black pepper, celery seed, lemon and orange peel (or powder made from lemon and orange peel), tarragon, fennel seed, white pepper, curry powder, hot pepper flakes, fresh garlic, and chives. Keep your eyes open for salt-free seasoning blends, too. Use vinegar (balsamic vinegar is particularly flavorful), lemon, and/or low-sodium tomato sauce—these acidic ingredients impart a piquant flavor to dishes that makes a nice alternative to salt.

There! Now you'll never have to say "Please pass the salt" again. Instead, let's talk about a nutrient over which there's often a good deal of controversy: protein. Read on, and you'll learn what you *really* need to know about this "building block of life."

CHAPTER 7

The Protein Paradox

Think of protein, and the very first things that probably come to mind are meat, eggs, milk, and cheese, and how healthy they're supposed to be: Didn't your parents urge you to drink plenty of milk? Didn't the football coach sit the team down to a steak before a big game? How about the all-American breakfast—bacon and eggs? It was once a virtual axiom that you stocked up on protein for energy and strength, and you got it from all the red meat, eggs, and dairy products you could squeeze into three square meals a day.

How times have changed! So many health-conscious people have come to realize that the traditional sources of protein are *not* as terrific as generations of doctors, nutritionists, and parents once made them out to be. But even those who know this much about diet and good nutrition are still worried about what—and how much—to eat instead. And if they ever tried to figure out how to mix and match plant proteins in order to end up with the right "complete" combination (which, as you'll soon learn, is completely unnecessary), they discovered how intimidating the whole process can be and perhaps decided that finding healthy sources of protein can sometimes seem like a lot more trouble than it's worth.

But *you'll* soon learn from our meal plans that you don't have to be intimidated, and that the Pritikin plan's approach to protein couldn't be simpler. (In fact, once your healthy kitchen is in full operation, you'll see firsthand that getting the right amount of protein from the right sources simply isn't a mystery at all.) Yet many people may still

91

wonder if it's *really* all right to say good-bye to all those generous servings of what they always thought was the best "brain food." So to address the lingering doubts, let's take a look at what protein really is. What role does it play in your body? How much do you really need? What are the best ways of getting it? Get ready to dispel some myths!

PROTEIN BASICS

Protein is a crucial component of every cell and of many of the chemicals needed for life. Your blood vessels, bones, skin, nerves, muscles, cartilage, lymph, and hair all contain protein, as do your enzymes, antibodies, and some of your hormones. You couldn't digest food without protein—and that's only one of the hundreds of vital bodily functions that depend on it (blood clotting, delivery of oxygen and nutrients to your body's cells, and defense against deadly bacteria are others). Only water (and sometimes fat) makes up a larger percentage of body weight.

Obviously, the fact that protein is *important* isn't a myth—it's a key player in virtually every part of the body—but the idea that you need to consume huge amounts of it couldn't be more wrong. The current Recommended Dietary Allowance for protein is .8 grams per kilogram (2.2 pounds) of body weight for adults, or 44 grams for the average woman, and 56 grams for the average man. Many Americans routinely eat 100 or more grams of protein a day, most of it from fatty animal sources. On the Pritikin Lifetime Eating Plan, on the other hand, men and women would have 50 to 75 grams of protein on a 2,000-calories-a-day plan—but this protein would come from nonfat dairy products, lean meat, lean poultry, fish, grains, vegetables, and legumes. On the Pritikin plan, a daily $3\frac{1}{2}$-ounce serving of fish, lean fowl, or lean meat will provide about half the average protein requirement, with the rest filled easily by legumes, grains, vegetables, fruits, and nonfat dairy foods low in fat and cholesterol (see Table 7-1).

To be utilized by the body, the large, complex molecules of protein in any food must first be broken down by the digestive tract into nitrogen-containing amino acids, protein's basic building blocks. Once digested and absorbed, the amino acids travel through the

TABLE 7-1
PROTEIN CONTENT, IN GRAMS, OF SELECTED FOODS ON THE PRITIKIN PLAN

Yogurt (1 cup)	13.0	Asparagus ($\frac{1}{2}$ cup cooked)	1.8
Egg white (1)	3.4	Spinach ($\frac{1}{2}$ cup cooked)	2.7
Skim milk (1 cup)	8.4	Broccoli (1 stalk)	3.6
Oatmeal ($\frac{1}{2}$ cup)	3.0	Cauliflower (1 cup raw)	2.7
Brown rice ($\frac{1}{3}$ cup)	1.5	Mushrooms (10 small)	2.7
Wheat bread (one slice)	2.4	Cantaloupe (1 cup)	1.3
Kidney beans ($\frac{1}{3}$ cup)	6.5	Apricots (4 medium)	2.0

bloodstream to wherever they're needed, and then regroup to form protein all over again. On its own, the human body can manufacture all but nine of the more than twenty amino acids it needs. These nine must be obtained in finished form from the protein foods we eat.

But obtaining these necessary amino acids in finished form does *not* mean overdosing on protein-rich foods—particularly animal protein—because a little protein goes a surprisingly long way. One indicator of whether you are getting enough protein is whether or not you are in "nitrogen balance"—that is, whether your body is retaining as much nitrogen, a product of protein metabolism, as it is excreting.

When people are switched from high- to low- or moderate-protein diets, it usually takes several weeks for them to adjust and reach a state of nitrogen balance again. But research by Walter Kempner, M.D., has shown that a 2,000-calorie-a-day diet supplying 93 percent of its calories from carbohydrates, 2.3 percent of its calories from fat, and only 4.7 percent of its calories from plant protein would in fact be enough to put you in a state of nitrogen balance within two or three months.[1]

Other studies have found that a diet of just 6 to 8 percent vegetable protein would put you back in nitrogen balance right away.[2] And since almost all the experimental protein-feeding studies conducted on humans to establish protein requirements have been very short in duration (as short as three to seven days), their results have often been misleading and may have overestimated the amounts we actually need.

One interesting thing we do know is that as a percentage of caloric intake, the protein requirement for human infants is at least two to three times higher than that for adults—yet protein accounts for only 6 to 7 percent of the calories in human breast milk, the preferred and superbly beneficial sole source of nutrition for the vast majority of American babies up to the age of six months today. Although the quality of this protein is uniquely beneficial for infants, it is interesting to point out that this is less than you'll find in a potato, most vegetables, grains, and even some fruits!

THE "INCOMPLETE-PROTEIN" MYTH

One of the most tenacious myths about protein is that the proteins derived from vegetables and grains are "incomplete," or of "poor quality," compared to those from animal sources. You've probably heard the familiar warning that the only way to obtain all the essential amino acids from these "incomplete" plant foods is to carefully combine various plant proteins, such as beans with grains, or seeds with grains. Faced with a choice between a steak and a library of mix-and-match instructions about unfamiliar foods, it's not surprising that many people just throw up their hands and choose the T-bone. The problem, however, is not that choosing the right protein is difficult. The problem is that these people are misinformed. The "incomplete plant food" argument just doesn't hold up. Here's why.

All plant foods, as grown, contain a combination of protein, fats, and carbohydrates. In this respect, whole grains and legumes are particularly nutritious: Not only are they ideal complex carbohydrates, rich in vitamins, minerals, and fiber, but they're also excellent sources of protein that contain small amounts of fat.

So why were they ever labeled "incomplete"? You can blame the rats—the laboratory rats that have been tested in protein experiments since the early 1900s. In early experiments (which were limited to rats), scientists noted that animals fed plant or vegetable proteins—grains, legumes, and greens—grew less rapidly than those fed the proteins found in meats, dairy foods, and eggs. When it was found that the amount of certain essential amino acids is lower in plant than in animal proteins, the plant proteins were labeled "incomplete." The findings of these laboratory-animal experiments were then flatly applied to humans, on the blind assumption that unless *we* ate sufficient amounts of animal protein, we'd suffer as badly as the rodents did.

You'll be happy to hear that, in experiments conducted on our own species, researchers have gathered far more accurate information about our protein requirements. Consider a few examples:

- Over a two-month period, a group of twenty- to twenty-seven-year-old men were put on diets equal in total calories, but different in protein source: On the first diet, 100 percent of the protein came from rice; on the second, 85 percent came from rice and 15 percent from chicken. In each case, only about 6.5 percent of the calories in the overall diet came from protein. Men eating the rice-only protein not only readily achieved a positive nitrogen balance, but they showed a *more positive* nitrogen balance than those who ate the rice-and-chicken meals![3]
- Two groups of young adults, on two equal-calorie diets, showed similar patterns: The protein source for the first group was exclusively eggs, while the second group's was a combination of eggs and potatoes (animal plus vegetable protein). The second group needed 36 percent less protein to achieve a positive nitrogen balance than those on the eggs alone![4]
- Another experiment clarifies that even for rapidly growing five- to fourteen-month-old babies there is no difference in the growth rate between those on all-cereal proteins and those on milk proteins.[5] And for those newborns and infants under six months whose sole food source is breast milk? Remember, human milk is only 6 to 7 percent protein, while rat's milk contains up to four times this amount. Compare the two: Human breast milk would be woefully inadequate for the newborn rat, yet human babies thrive on it. It's clear that basing our protein requirements on those of rats just doesn't make any sense.

The great protein myth builds on this basic error: It presumes that because vegetable proteins contain small amounts of certain essential amino acids and are thus "inferior" in a diet for rats, they must be painstakingly combined to "completion" for humans to meet their everyday requirements. But in fact, if you follow the Pritikin plan guidelines—regardless of calorie level—you don't have to combine *any* proteins, even if you're a strict vegetarian. (When she revised her best-selling book ten years after it was published, Frances Moore Lappé, author of *Diet for a Small Planet*, corrected herself for having promoted the myth that vegetable proteins must be carefully combined to meet daily requirements.)

When consumed in adequate quantities and varieties, all combinations of all plant foods, including vegetables, legumes, grains, and fruits, naturally contain plenty of all the essential amino acids (or protein "building blocks") to satisfy your daily needs. This includes the nine essential amino acids (out of the total of twenty-three) which the body cannot make on its own. With its enormous variety of "grown" foods as well as its small amounts of animal proteins, the Pritikin Lifetime Eating Plan provides all amino acids—both essential and nonessential—in abundance.

Some foods do provide lower amounts of certain amino acids than others, but again, if you are consuming adequate calories from healthy sources, you don't have to worry. One study showed that a diet where 90–95 percent of the protein came from white flour and the remaining 5–10 percent came from fruits and vegetables was adequate to maintain nitrogen balance.[6]

THE DANGERS OF EXCESS

Now that we've seen how much less animal protein (and protein in general) we need to consume than we thought we did, it's natural to wonder if there's any danger in consuming too much. The answer is, in a word, "Absolutely."

Too much protein can be a problem in several ways. For one thing, animal protein foods too often contain excess fat and cholesterol (as in the foods our parents once innocently urged us to eat, like eggs, red meat, and cheese), which increase the risk of a variety of chronic diseases. In addition, researchers have shown that even purified animal protein, devoid of cholesterol, when substituted for vegetable protein, is associated with a significant rise in serum cholesterol. Much more research is needed in this area, but it appears to be another reason to avoid eating excessive animal protein.[7]

For humans, among the worst of the diseases associated with high-fat animal protein are probably certain cancers, including those of the breast, colon, rectum, and endometrium. Interestingly, some scientists believe that the protein in these foods may be as much to blame as the fat: According to a report by the National Research

Council, fat is not the only thing that promotes tumor growth. At the very least, the cancer-stimulating effects of excess fat and protein may turn out to reinforce each other.[8]

And, of course, there's no escaping the horribly high fat content of most animal protein: Whole-milk products, egg yolks, and red meat will make *you* fat if you don't carefully restrict your calories (which will, in turn, on this kind of diet, make you chronically hungry!). The percentage of fat in "high-protein" foods such as meat and cheese is astonishing—they actually contain a much greater proportion of fat than protein! For example, a chuck steak is about 66 percent fat and only 33 percent protein; regular cheddar cheese gets about 74 percent of its calories from fat and only 24 percent from protein; and 64 percent of the calories in an egg come from fat, while 30 percent come from protein! To top it all off, any surplus protein not used by the body for either energy or repair will end up being stored as fat.

All protein also breaks down in the body into potentially toxic nitrogen by-products such as ammonia and urea, which need to be flushed out with large amounts of water. Another by-product of the breakdown is sulfur, which is excreted as sulfate. But the body must draw on its reserves of alkaline minerals such as calcium and magnesium to neutralize the sulfate. That means there are two potential side effects of excess animal protein (or even vegetable protein, for that matter): the loss of bone minerals (perhaps posing the risk of osteoporosis),[9] and dehydration. One study showed that even a daily 2,300-milligram supplement of calcium could not compensate for the mineral-robbing effects of excess protein,[10] and many other studies have documented the adverse effects of excessive protein intake on calcium loss as well.[11-13]

BEWARE OF HIGH-PROTEIN WEIGHT-LOSS DIETS

What about all those "lose 10 pounds in four days" high-protein diets? At the very least, can't you rely on them to take off a few fast pounds at the beginning of a more "sensible" diet?

The trouble with high-protein diets aimed at quick weight loss is that the weight you lose consists primarily of water and glycogen (carbohydrates stored in the liver and muscles). Once you go off these diets and start eating more carbohydrates again, your body retains water and glycogen more stubbornly to compensate for the previous shortage, leading to a weight-gain "rebound." Even worse, because these high-protein diets are often too low in both carbohydrates and calories, the protein you eat must be used mostly for energy. This means that the protein needed for building and repairing body tissues may be drawn from your own lean muscle. So after you lose weight, you may be left with a higher proportion of fat to muscle than before you started.

If your goal is to slim down, this cycle could be self-defeating. Burdened with a higher proportion of fat to muscle, your body won't burn calories as quickly, since fat uses up energy more slowly than lean tissue. That means you'll appear flabbier and less "defined" than before, even if you end up weighing less (since muscle is slightly heavier than fat). In the more likely event that you gain back your lost weight ("quick" protein diets deliver only short-term results), you're less likely to lose it the next time around. What's worse, by raising levels of serum cholesterol and uric acid, these diets do exactly what excess protein does: They increase your risk for serious illness. So not only are high-protein weight-loss diets generally ineffective over the long haul, they're actually hazardous to your health.

WHAT ABOUT PROTEIN FOR POWER?

This is another persistent—and perhaps the most dangerous— protein falsehood: that protein is the very best nutrient for athletes.

These "extra-active" people were once thought to need prodigious amounts of protein for muscle power and endurance, and in many minds the notion still persists. But protein is a demanding, dehydrating form of energy that depletes the body of up to seven times more water per calorie than do carbohydrates—hardly an asset for peak performance! But a high-carbohydrate eating plan will provide *more* endurance than one that's high in protein: This kind of eating plan helps keep muscles constantly loaded with glycogen, the storage form of carbohydrate, which releases a steady surge of energy. And remember, excess protein never turns into muscle—only into fat.

By increasing your intake of unrefined carbohydrates and at the same time reducing your reliance on fatty animal protein foods, you'll automatically decrease the amount of cholesterol circulating in your bloodstream. Too much fat can aggregate red blood cells and block tiny capillaries, leading to oxygen-starved muscles.[14] What's more, the brain's *only* fuel (unless you're on a long-term fast, which we do *not* recommend!) is glucose, so a high-carbohydrate, low-fat diet will give you the mental alertness and clarity you need to sustain any strenuous physical performance. The bottom line? You just don't need animal protein for strength or endurance.

Perhaps the world's most dramatic example of an eating plan that can lead to peak performance can be seen in Mexico's frequently studied Tarahumara Indians, who consume a diet of complex carbohydrates and vegetable protein (corn, squash, beans, peas, and fruit) plus a small amount of animal protein about once a month. Their national sport, a kickball game which has made them world famous, involves running tremendous distances nonstop—175 miles in about 48 hours—a feat that makes most 26.2-mile marathons look like a stroll around the block! Equally inspiring is the virtual absence of obesity, heart disease, hypertension, and diabetes in their population. Close at the figurative heels of the Tarahumara Indians are a number of top world-class athletes, including many Olympic contenders, who are very often proponents of a low-fat, high-carbohydrate diet like the Pritikin plan.

While protein needs increase somewhat during pregnancy and breast-feeding, as well as when you're under unusual stress, they do not increase enormously, as is commonly believed. You certainly don't have to increase your intake of animal foods to handle the greater need; since *all* foods contain protein, any additional requirement can be met simply by increasing your calorie intake of the *right* foods.

The same applies to any prolonged, vigorous exercise: Just eating more complex carbohydrates such as beans and grains, which generally are rich sources of vegetable protein, will easily help you meet any increased demand for protein. And while it's true that the human body uses up somewhat more protein than normal after surgery or during times of physical stress, only severe physical trauma (such as suffering major burns) significantly increases the need for protein. Even then, a large dose of protein doesn't have to be accompanied by fat, as it is in most of the animal protein foods you *used* to think were good for you.

PROTEIN POINTERS

Just as you don't need to eat a lot of protein, there isn't a lot of complicated information to remember about it, either. This is all it takes:

- *All foods, as grown, contain protein,* so if you eat the proper variety in sufficient quantity, it's easy to meet your protein needs. A varied diet that includes whole grains, beans, fruits, and vegetables can easily meet an adult's protein requirements.
- *The healthiest sources of protein are legumes, whole grains, vegetables, and nonfat dairy products* in proper quantities—*not* high-fat meats, full-fat dairy products, and eggs.
- *A little protein goes a long way.* Only 10 to 15 percent of your daily calories need to come from protein, and excess protein calories *always* convert into body fat.
- *Many sources of animal protein are high in fat,* and can therefore increase your risk of certain diseases related to fat consumption.
- *High-protein quick-weight-loss diets are bad news*—they don't work in the long run and they're hazardous to your health.
- *For peak performance, unrefined carbohydrates are the best fuel,* not animal protein.

That's it! As we said, the Pritikin plan's approach to protein couldn't be simpler. Nor, in fact, could our approach to what just may be today's most talked-about dietary bonus—fiber. Once you get the inside scoop on this essential component of a truly healthy eating plan, you may be surprised to learn that it can do even *more* for you than you may have thought!

CHAPTER 8

The Fiber Factor

How much fiber do you need? To judge from the storm of publicity it's received, from all the fiber supplements you can buy, and from the cereals, soups, and other foods that all promise "More fiber!" you may wonder if anything less than a diet of twigs and hay will do. Actually, it's good news that in the past decade public consciousness has been raised about the importance of fiber in the diet. What's even better news is the fact that, as long as you stay on the Pritikin Lifetime Eating Plan, you'll get all the fiber you need, without supplements. Sharon B. remembers the days when she added two or three tablespoons of bran to her breakfast cereal every morning. That was before she discovered the Pritikin plan. "Now," she says, "I don't have to add anything. I'm getting all the fiber benefits I can get just by following the Lifetime Eating Plan."

She—and you—will continue to get these benefits because Pritikin meals automatically provide ample amounts of both soluble *and* insoluble fiber (you'll learn about these distinctions soon); quality and quantity are built into the foods themselves. Sharon's longtime habit of adding fiber to foods that were too high in fat and refined sugar had given her a false sense of security. When a checkup showed that she had elevated cholesterol and triglycerides, she realized that the foods she had been eating every day were harmful to her body—and that adding a lot of bran to her cereal, while it may have had some benefit, obviously wasn't a complete answer.

Nutrition authorities now agree that it's better to obtain fiber naturally, from a wide variety of whole, unprocessed foods, than to add

101

it as a separate ingredient (in the form of guar gum, fiber laxatives, or wheat bran, for example) to an otherwise fiber-deficient eating plan.

Americans eat about 10 to 15 grams of fiber a day, and current recommendations from the National Cancer Institute advise increasing that total to about 20 to 30 grams.[1] The Pritikin Lifetime Eating Plan provides at least 35 grams of fiber a day—which, as you'll see shortly, seems to be the optimal amount for healthy individuals. This abundance is simply a dividend of menus rich in whole grains, legumes, vegetables, and fruits.

WHAT IS "FIBER"?

Found in all plant foods, "fiber" refers to those parts that cannot be broken down by the enzymes and secretions in our digestive tracts. Basically, fiber is derived from the material that helps give plants their upright shape and structure, or from substances that are mixed with plant starches.

The different varieties of fiber (chiefly cellulose, hemicellulose, lignin, pectin, gums, and mucilages) belong to one of two major categories, each with its own special properties. *Insoluble fiber,* the coarse, gritty kind that doesn't dissolve in even the hottest liquid, is probably the one you know best in the form of wheat bran. It's found in all whole grains, and to a lesser extent in beans, vegetables, and fruits. *Soluble fiber,* soft and gummy by comparison, is found in oat bran, beans and peas (legumes), oats, barley, fruits, carrots, sweet potatoes, yams, and other vegetables.

For the longest time, fiber (once known more graphically as "roughage") was regarded as a cure for constipation—period. After all, this was the folk wisdom handed down by many well-meaning grandparents who urged a daily dose of a food like beans or hot wheat cereal to help keep us "regular." Our grandparents were, in fact, right.

In the 1970s, fiber became front-page news. Drs. Denis Burkitt and Hugh Trowell and other researchers noted that populations eating diets rich in fiber and low in animal foods suffered from very few of the familiar Western ills, such as colon-rectal cancer, diverticulosis, heart disease, obesity, and diabetes.[2] While their diets were also lower in fat, cholesterol, and salt and higher in carbohydrates than those of most Americans, the abundance of fiber they consumed was believed to offer additional protection.

A VARIETY OF BENEFITS

Today we know that your diet should include adequate amounts of both soluble and insoluble fiber for maximum benefit—a balance assured by eating a variety of foods from each group on the Pritikin Lifetime Eating Plan. Because it's spongelike, the insoluble fiber found in wheat bran and grains absorbs many times its own weight in liquid, making stools larger and softer. Propelled more quickly by the added bulk, the digested food has less time to deposit chemical impurities and cancer-promoting compounds on the intestinal wall. Also, the generous amount of water absorbed by the fiber dilutes any potential carcinogens in the intestines or stool itself. This may be one reason that diets high in bran and cereal fiber are associated with markedly lower rates of colon cancer.

Consistently softer, bulkier stools also mean that diverticulosis, appendicitis, hemorrhoids, and varicose veins are far less likely, since all these conditions may result in part from rectal straining, higher intra-abdominal pressure, and slower transit time within the large intestine.

Soluble fiber helps to lower blood cholesterol. For example, oat bran, beans, carrots, and other foods containing soluble fiber have been shown to reduce serum levels of LDL ("bad") cholesterol and of total cholesterol.[3] These fibers are believed to link up with bile acids (compounds that originally derived from cholesterol stores in the liver), escorting them out of the body. And by slowing the absorption of carbohydrates, they may help stabilize blood sugar levels and reduce the body's wide swings in insulin secretion—which makes them useful in controlling diabetes. Studies with both healthy individuals and diabetics have shown that when soluble fiber is included in a high-carbohydrate meal, insulin and blood sugar levels do not rise as high as they do when the fiber is removed.[4]

As for other benefits, insoluble fiber may discourage digestive-tract disorders such as irritable-bowel syndrome and reduce the likelihood of gallstones.

HOW FIBER FIGHTS FAT

On an eating plan rich in carbohydrates and fiber from grains, vegetables, legumes, and fruits, you will automatically be consuming little fat, refined sugar, and cholesterol. This not only protects you from major diseases, but also provides built-in weight control. Because many high-fiber foods require a good deal more chewing than refined foods and animal products, you're less likely to rush through meals and overeat. Bulky, water-absorbing, fiber-rich foods also swell inside your stomach and delay gastric emptying, making you feel satisfied and full. What's more, they offer plenty of carbohydrates, protein, vitamins, and minerals in exchange for very few calories.

High-fiber foods are used directly for energy and are less likely than fats to be stored as extra pounds (but they will be, of course, if they're eaten in excess; you'll learn about this in Chapter 9 when we discuss the benefits of unrefined carbohydrates). Foods in their natural state (or as close to it as possible), like a fresh apple or a baked potato, contain soluble and insoluble fiber, along with vitamins, minerals, essential fatty acids, and other components. The presence of both soluble and insoluble fiber in a meal may also reduce somewhat the number of calories you absorb from other foods you eat. And, as you'll also learn in Chapter 9, some studies have shown that soluble fibers may aid in weight loss by reducing insulin levels and appetite and therefore calorie intake and fat storage.[5]

HIGH-FIBER FOODS

One obvious advantage of foods rich in fiber is that there are so many of them—and you can combine and cook them in nearly endless ways (see Table 8-1 for a sampling). The whole range of grains, legumes, vegetables, and fruits you have at your command and the endless number of casseroles, salads, side dishes, soups, stews, and even desserts into which they can be made promise astounding versatility.

All the whole grains are excellent sources of fiber: whole wheat, bulgur, barley, millet, oats, whole rye, triticale, brown and basmati

TABLE 8-1
FIBER CONTENT OF SELECTED FOODS

Food	Serving	Insoluble Fiber (grams)	Soluble Fiber (grams)	Calories
GRAINS				
Bread, whole-wheat	1 slice	1.2	.3	61
Barley, pearled, dry	2 Tbsp.	1.0	1.5	97
Cornmeal, whole-grain	2 Tbsp.	1.8	.2	54
Oat bran, dry	$\frac{1}{3}$ cup	2.2	2.0	90
Oats, regular, dry	$\frac{1}{3}$ cup	1.5	1.3	100
FRUITS				
Apple, with skin	1	2.1	.9	80
Banana	$\frac{1}{2}$ medium	.7	.3	46
Dates, dried	2	1.2	.4	50
Figs, dried	1 medium	2.9	3.7	55
Strawberries	$1\frac{1}{4}$ cup	2.0	1.2	60
Orange	1 small	.9	.3	40
VEGETABLES				
Broccoli, cooked	$\frac{1}{2}$ cup	1.1	.9	28
Brussels sprouts, cooked	$\frac{1}{2}$ cup	2.3	1.6	30
Cabbage, Chinese, cooked	$\frac{1}{2}$ cup	1.2	1.6	30
Carrots, cooked	$\frac{1}{2}$ cup	1.2	1.1	21
Cauliflower, cooked	$\frac{1}{2}$ cup	1.1	.5	14
Corn, cooked	$\frac{1}{2}$ cup	2.7	.2	71
Kale, cooked	$\frac{1}{2}$ cup	1.4	1.4	20
Peas, young green, cooked	$\frac{1}{2}$ cup	3.0	1.1	57
Onion, cooked	$\frac{1}{2}$ cup	1.4	.8	32
Potato, white, baked	$\frac{1}{2}$ medium	1.0	.9	73
Yam, cooked	$\frac{1}{2}$ medium	1.4	1.5	80
BEANS				
Kidney beans, cooked	$\frac{1}{2}$ cup	3.3	2.5	115
Lima beans, cooked	$\frac{1}{2}$ cup	3.2	1.2	64
Pinto beans, cooked	$\frac{1}{2}$ cup	3.3	2.0	114
Lentils, cooked	$\frac{1}{2}$ cup	1.1	.9	58
Peas, black-eyed, cooked	$\frac{1}{2}$ cup	6.8	4.5	145

Source: James W. Anderson, *Plant Fiber in Foods.* Lexington, Kentucky: HCF Diabetes Research Foundation, 1986; James W. Anderson, "Dietary fiber content of selected foods," *American Journal of Clinical Nutrition,* 47:440–447, 1988; and the Quaker Oats Analytical Laboratory.

rice, whole-grain cornmeal, and the more exotic, highly nutritious new imports like amaranth and quinoa. (Many ethnic cuisines, such as Mexican, Italian, Oriental, and Middle Eastern, are terrific and inexpensive sources of the right kinds of carbohydrates, protein, vitamins, minerals—and fiber.) Legumes such as garbanzos, red kidney beans, black-eyed peas, and lentils (to name only a few of the scores of varieties available) offer the double benefits of soluble fiber and vegetable protein.

Among the vegetables, fiber-packed favorites include broccoli, brussels sprouts, cabbage, carrots, corn, eggplant, kale, peppers, potatoes, squash, and spinach. As for fruits, fresh apples and pears, as well as raspberries, top the list for fiber, along with citrus fruits and all other kinds of berries. But all other fruits and vegetables contain these fibers, too, so be sure to eat a wide variety.

Unfortunately, most of our omnipresent "convenience" foods—which make up more than 50 percent of this country's daily diet—are virtually devoid of fiber and typically high in fat, sodium, and sugar. This is no coincidence, as you'll soon see: In highly processed carbohydrates, the more highly processed the food item, the more likely that it lacks essentials for your health. So remember, to ensure maximum nutrients and fiber, eat foods in as close to their natural state as possible.

CAN YOU OVERDOSE ON FIBER?

Some researchers claim that excess fiber may interfere with the absorption of certain nutrients, such as calcium, iron, and zinc. But while several studies have shown that adopting a natural high-fiber regimen causes a small drop in the absorption of certain minerals at first, other research suggests that this effect is only temporary since the body adapts after a few weeks and returns to its previous normal levels.[6] In any case, since natural whole foods are better sources of most vitamins and minerals, a small drop in absorption is of little import.

Phytates (phytic acid), a component of fiber, have often been singled out as the factor responsible for this transient decline, but research by the Nutrition Institute of the U.S. Department of Agriculture has not shown this to be true.[7] Another study, this one performed by Dr. James W. Anderson, chief of endocrinology at the University of Kentucky Medical Center, measured the effects of a diet consisting of 50 to 70 grams of dietary fiber—from vegetables, whole grains, legumes, fruits, and $\frac{2}{3}$ cup of oat bran a day—on a group of diabetics for an average of twenty-one months[8] (some were tested for up to fifty-one months). The group did not show any drop in blood levels of calcium, phosphorus, iron, or even magnesium, a mineral in which diabetics may be deficient. In fact, research at a Pritikin Longevity Center showed that people following this type of eating plan for as long as *five years* had normal levels of vitamins and minerals. In some cases, these levels were higher than in those people consuming a more traditional diet.[9] It appears clear that people who eat even relatively large amounts of dietary fiber remain in a consistent state of mineral balance (that is, they retain as many minerals as they lose), without showing signs of nutritional deficiency.

So, can you overdose on fiber? You can probably take too much as a supplement, just as you can take anything to the point of its not helping you anymore—or even to the point of toxicity. But you will derive *optimal* benefit by consuming what is provided naturally in the foods recommended on the Pritikin Lifetime Eating Plan: Unless you have certain acute intestinal disorders such as diverticulitis, or an exacerbation of an inflammatory bowel disease such as ulcerative colitis or Crohn's disease, if you're following the Pritikin plan you simply don't have to worry about consuming too much—and you certainly don't have to worry about not getting enough!

A DELICATE SUBJECT

Some people find that when they switch to high-fiber meals they experience increased flatulence—and, in fact, you may experience this temporarily or occasionally on the Pritikin eating plan. To keep this problem to a minimum, bear the following suggestions in mind:

- Avoid overeating at any one meal. Large high-fiber meals, because they speed intestinal transit time, increase the number of undigested proteins and carbohydrates reaching the colon. This tends to increase gas, which results from the action of intestinal bacteria on this undigested material.

- Use whole-grain products, and limit or eliminate wheat bran and other concentrated fiber foods.
- Soak legumes and discard soaking water before cooking.
- Choose more lightly cooked vegetables (preferably steamed, parboiled, or stir-"fried") and fewer raw vegetables.
- Avoid combining several gassy foods in one meal. Raw vegetable salad, bean soup, broccoli, and whole-grain crackers would be a meal likely to cause gas—even for those accustomed to a high-fiber diet.

A little gas is perfectly normal! If you do end up experiencing some bloating or flatulence, just remember that it may diminish or simply disappear in time—and that it will be vastly outweighed by the long-term benefits you'll derive from better health and increased energy.

ABOUT FIBER SUPPLEMENTS

If your diet is composed of high-fat, highly processed foods, sprinkling a little bran on your cereal is not the ideal way to get an adequate amount of fiber. Neither will going to the other extreme help you: Adding 40 to 60 grams of supplemental fiber in powder or pill form would be excessive and could possibly lead to nutrient-absorption problems. In fact, the American Institute for Cancer Research recommends getting fiber from foods rather than from fiber supplements.[10]

While today's new focus on fiber is encouraging, some health professionals and best-selling diet books have unfortunately chosen to recommend fiber supplements instead of suggesting changes in basic eating habits. This practice may be self-defeating, because it's rather like choosing to take an antidote instead of eliminating the poison itself. Meals that are high in fat and cholesterol and low in unrefined carbohydrates put us at risk for chronic diseases and obesity—and fiber supplements are not the magical correction for these imbalances. It's true that adding fiber will help lower two risk factors associated with high-fat diets—high cholesterol and colon cancer—but fiber supplements will not address the other health risks associated with a high-fat diet.

Fiber supplements are also a poor substitute for real food— unprocessed, fiber-rich carbohydrates with all their nutritional advantages. What's more, they are expensive and can easily lull people into complacency ("*My* diet is healthy—I add fiber to it every day, don't I?"). With growing numbers of people becoming more conscious of the benefits of fiber, health authorities would be better advised to help them improve their daily diets instead of offering them yet another drugstore prescription.

Of course, once you're following the Pritikin plan, you won't have to worry about *any* of this at all! For followers of the Pritikin plan, it couldn't be simpler: The best way to consume fiber is from unrefined, unprocessed whole grains, vegetables, and fruits—and you'll get *all* you need from the Pritikin Lifetime Eating Plan.

Now let's move on to the centerpiece of our nutritional plan: carbohydrates. You've heard from the outset how important they are, and all the valuable knowledge you've gained in the last five chapters will soon help you understand why.

CHAPTER 9

Carbohydrates: Food for Life

You'll see from the briefest glance at a menu from the Pritikin program that the old meat-and-potatoes approach to dinner (with meat clearly more important and potatoes as just a "side dish") has been reversed. Once thought of merely as "fillers," potatoes, grains, beans, and other carbohydrates are now being valued as meals in themselves, whether it's rice pilaf, pasta, or an Oriental stir-"fry." By emphasizing these foods, the Pritikin Lifetime Eating Plan does more than change your perspective about what you put on your plate: It reduces your risk of serious, life-shortening diseases and virtually guarantees safe, effective weight loss without calorie counting.

But many otherwise nutrition-conscious eaters—and you may have been one of them before you learned about a low-fat, high-complex-carbohydrate diet—still cling to the notion that carbohydrates in general are fattening. Weren't we always taught that potatoes and spaghetti are fattening? The consensus was generally that, yes, breads, cereals, pasta, and other starchy foods had nutritional value, but they were too high in calories, so we couldn't eat much of them.

The fact is that carbohydrates (especially unrefined carbohydrates) not only ensure long-term health and well-being, but they're also an *essential* part of a permanent *weight-loss* eating plan. Here's why.

COMPLEX OR SIMPLE?

Nature's most abundant sources of energy, carbohydrates—starches and sugars—are made up of the elements carbon, hydrogen, and

110

oxygen. Carbohydrates supply approximately 4 calories per gram, and are considered the best providers of fuel for the human body.

Technically, starches are complex carbohydrates, and sugars are simple carbohydrates. But actually they're both made up entirely of sugar molecules. What's the difference, then, between "complex" and "simple"? Complex carbohydrates, which include the starches found in vegetables, legumes, and grains, are composed not of one or two but of hundreds to thousands of sugar (glucose) molecules chained together. Simple carbohydrates, such as those found in table sugar or in fruit, are either monosaccharides or disaccharides (which means they consist of either one or two sugar molecules). All unrefined carbohydrates—simple and complex—provide us with energy, fiber, and very important nutrients.

REFINED OR UNREFINED?

When you eat a potato or an apple, you get a slower, steadier supply of energy than you do if you drink apple juice or eat instant mashed potatoes, which are more refined products. In their unrefined form (as a potato, corn on the cob, or a whole, fresh apple), both simple and complex carbohydrates are used by the body as it needs them, instead of giving the body too much energy too soon, as the refined carbohydrates in white bread or a cola drink do.

Think of your body as a fuel-burning stove, and your choice of fuel as a pile of tissue paper or a stack of logs. Toss in the tissue paper and you'll get a momentary burst of flame—but burn the logs and you'll have heat for hours. Similarly, unrefined carbohydrates will give you longer-lasting fuel, as well as protein, minerals, trace elements, essential fatty acids, and generous amounts of vitamins, such as the B-complex vitamins. With their high fiber content, unrefined carbohydrates will also help satisfy your appetite and give you a feeling of satiety—as well as provide you with all the benefits only fiber has.

Highly refined and processed foods are a relatively recent phenomenon in Western civilization. The typical Western diet now eliminates valuable fiber and nutrients and overconcentrates sugars and starches to create foods that are calorically more dense. (In addition to providing unneeded calories, refined carbohydrates can upset the body's blood sugar balance.) Consider refined white flour or table sugar—and how radically altered each of them is from its original state. The flour has been depleted of its vitamin-rich germ, most of its essential fatty acids and minerals, and the outer, fibrous shell; similarly, refined sugar is an even longer way from the natural raw sugar beet and sugarcane, which are actually very high in fiber and in vitamins and minerals as well.

Eating vegetables, whole grains, legumes, and fruits is a lot more like the way human beings ate before "civilized" Western countries established their standards of what constitutes "good eating." Our long, meandering digestive tracts, the structure of our teeth, the enzyme content of our saliva, the fact that we have hands (rather than claws), our metabolic makeup, our kidneys—all unchanged for thousands of years—are best suited to the primarily plant- and fruit-based menus of early humans, and these menus form the prototype of the Pritikin eating plan.

As recently as 1900, most of the Western world still derived nearly 70 percent of its protein from plant—not animal—sources, but the picture is completely reversed today. Dietary mainstays are now meats, poultry, fish, eggs, and cheese, as well as refined, processed foods high in fats and sugar. It's no coincidence that the rate of chronic, debilitating diseases—including obesity—has dramatically increased. Digestive disturbances and a host of other everyday complaints (which we often think are "inevitable" and we'll simply have to live with) also seem to be strongly linked to our errant life-style and eating habits. What we've discovered (and what new data continue to support) is that on our body's original meal plan—a diet rich in unrefined carbohydrates, low in fats, and moderate in protein (protein derived mostly from plant sources)—we can achieve a more lasting vigor and protect ourselves from a catalog of degenerative diseases like cancer and heart disease, and from less serious but annoying ills such as constipation and gallstones.

PEAK PERFORMANCE

More than simply preventing or correcting those ills, an eating plan based on unrefined carbohydrates can also help boost our health to our genetic potential and give those of us who pursue sports a real competitive edge. Top world-class athletes in many sports are now embracing a low-fat, high-carbohydrate program for peak performance, stamina, and strength—athletes like Dave Scott, Scott Tinley, and Scott Molina, who placed first, second, and fourth, respectively, in the grueling Hawaii Ironman Triathlon in the fall of 1982 (this triathlon consists of a 2.4-mile ocean swim, a 112-mile bicycle race, and a 26.2-mile marathon run). In the 1982 competition, Dave Scott captured first place with a new record time that was sixteen minutes faster than his own best time—an exciting breakthrough victory. His Pritikin eating plan, he felt, probably contributed to his outstanding triathlon performance. The increase in muscle and liver glycogen (stored energy) that resulted from his high-carbohydrate eating regimen enabled him to train for five to eight hours a day and to compete at world-class level. In 1983, 1984, 1986, and 1987 Dave Scott again led the pack in the Ironman—and in 1984 he shattered his own course record by more than ten minutes.

The astonishing endurance and success of athletes like these are eloquent proof that a diet high in unrefined carbohydrates is a diet of high-performance foods. But why are unrefined simple and complex carbohydrates the best and most efficient source of energy for athletes—and for the rest of us? Why do they supply optimal energy for our billions of active cells, including those that power our muscles, brain, and nervous system?

THE PERFECT FUEL

Unlike proteins, carbohydrates burn "clean." After the body breaks them down into usable units (molecules of sugar, or glucose), only carbon dioxide and water remain—perfectly harmless end products that we excrete easily through our lungs when we breathe. Any carbohydrates not utilized for fuel are stored in the liver and muscles in the form of glycogen. If a diet is very low in carbohydrates, the body is forced to rely more on fat and protein for energy. But fats burn inefficiently on very-low-carbohydrate diets and leave behind potentially toxic residues called ketones that turn the blood more acidic and interfere with normal body functions. Protein is less undesirable as an energy source, too, since it leaves behind potentially hazardous nitrogen and sulfur wastes that put extra stress on the kidneys as they perform their disposal function.

Protein is the body's major building and repair material, a chief constituent of everything from our muscles and bones to the enzymes that control all our chemical reactions. Protein is present in all our cells, but we need to eat only a *moderate* amount of it. (For one thing, some amino acids—they're the building blocks of proteins—are converted into body fat more readily than carbohydrates, so you might gain weight more quickly from eating excess amounts of certain proteins than excess amounts of carbohydrates.[1]) But our bodies need to have carbohydrates replenished in greater quantities and more often.

Fats are the most calorically concentrated foods you can eat, supplying at least 9 calories per gram. We say "at least" 9 calories since a recent animal study by Dr. Mark Hegsted, a noted Harvard University nutritionist, found that fat is in fact "worth" about 11 calories per gram inside the body.[2] (That would make fat, in terms of calories, nearly three times as concentrated as protein or carbohydrates, each of which provides 4 calories per gram.) According to Dr. Hegsted and other researchers, because dietary fat's chemical structure is essentially the same as body fat's, it is far easier (because it takes less energy) for the body to convert dietary fat into body fat than to change either carbohydrates or protein into body fat.

While fat is readily stored as fuel in our fat cells, the same is not true of carbohydrates or protein: The body has to work harder and use up more energy to store an equivalent number of calories from carbohydrates or protein as fat. If excess carbohydrates are eaten, the liver will convert them into fat, which is sent through the blood as VLDL triglycerides (see Chapter 5) and stored in fat cells. But about 25 percent of these carbohydrate calories never get converted into fat—they're burned in the conversion process.

Carbohydrates also provide the brain with its primary fuel. Unlike muscles, the brain does not burn either protein or fat for energy (except after prolonged fasting): Under normal circumstances glucose (blood sugar) is its primary food. This blood glucose comes mostly from glycogen stored in the liver.

TIME-RELEASED ENERGY

As we've said, in general, the less refined the carbohydrate, the more gradually its energy is released. Gradual release keeps blood sugar levels relatively stable and prevents the sharp fluctuations that lead to elevated insulin levels and aggravate problems with blood sugar regulation. Since insulin promotes fat storage, elevated levels of it may in turn promote greater fat storage. Higher insulin levels may also promote sodium retention and an increase in blood pressure. (You can see how closely interrelated the body's functions are—and why no *one* dietary element, like salt for high blood pressure or cholesterol for atherosclerosis, is solely responsible for disease.)

When Western-style diets are adopted by such groups as Australian aborigines or Pima Indians—who had previously depended on natural high-carbohydrate, low-fat diets—these populations develop the same diseases that we get, such as obesity, diabetes, hypertension, and gallstones. Typical Western diets have a demonstrably negative effect on health! Obesity and blood sugar abnormalities, including diabetes, were virtually unknown among the Australian aborigines and Pima Indians before they adopted Western-style foods, but they are now common. This is true also of populations in Micronesia.[3]

Indeed, populations throughout the world whose foods are high in unrefined carbohydrates and low in fats show a near absence of the degenerative disease patterns now linked to the typical Western diet. But when people from these populations move to areas where people eat as Americans do today, they may develop a host of chronic disorders from which they were previously protected by a natural-food diet.

THE WEIGHT-LOSS REWARD

You already know that a diet high in unrefined carbohydrates can enhance weight loss, if that's what you're after. One reason for this is that carbohydrates are such a clean-burning fuel: The body's capacity to store carbohydrates is limited, so they are less likely to be stockpiled as body fat, the way excess dietary fat is. And there's also the fact that you *feel* fuller after eating carbohydrates.

At Cornell University, Dr. Lauren Lissner examined the effects of varying the dietary fat in her subjects' diets. All the subjects were encouraged to eat as much food as they wanted, and all the food offered to them was judged to be equally palatable. Dr. Lissner and her colleagues found that the subjects automatically ate 600 to 700 fewer calories per day on the low-fat (15 to 20 percent fat calories) high-carbohydrate diet than on the high-fat (45 to 50 percent fat calories) diet, and the participants found the low-fat food just as satisfying. Not surprisingly, the subjects on the low-fat diet were losing weight and those on the high-fat diet were gaining weight.[4] This study obviously supports what we at the Pritikin Longevity Centers have found: that you'll consume fewer calories and lose weight on the low-fat, high-carbohydrate Lifetime Eating Plan— *without going hungry.*

To sum up, foods rich in carbohydrates in their whole or minimally processed state are the very best for your body. And most are also nutritional bargains: Naturally satisfying and low in fat, they are generous providers of vitamins, minerals, trace elements, essential fatty acids, protein, fiber, and energy in return for much less fat. But of the refined carbohydrates—both simple and complex—that still predominate in American diets today, even the ones that are "enriched" (such as white bread and presweetened breakfast cereals) have far fewer of most of their original nutrients, and little if any of the fiber of their whole, natural counterparts.

WHAT YOU NEED TO KNOW ABOUT SUGAR

The most plentiful of the refined carbohydrates are the sugars, which appear under an assortment of names and variations (you'll learn to recognize many of them after you take our "label-reading course" in Chapter 12): glucose, fructose, sucrose, maltose, corn syrup, corn sugar, maple sugar and maple syrup, invert sugar, and molasses. All of these provide a 4-calorie-per-gram dose of rapidly absorbed calories—and, with the exception of molasses, little or nothing else of nutritional value. However, while they may not be rich in basic nutrients, sugars themselves are not harmful if eaten in small amounts (although excess sugar can lead to unstable blood sugar levels, dental cavities, and, possibly, other consequences).

The excess fat, cholesterol, and sodium in foods are far more serious threats to health. In fact, most people who are labeled—or label themselves—"hypoglycemic" achieve normal blood sugar levels when they adopt a low-fat, high-fiber diet. Their blood sugar levels may soar and then swoop way down after they eat too much sugar, but this doesn't necessarily mean they're metabolically predisposed to hypoglycemia: They're simply reacting normally to an overconsumption of refined sugar! And as for diabetes, many people have long believed that sugar is the culprit—however, as you learned in Chapter 4, excessive caloric intake associated with dietary fat probably plays a more critical role in the major type of this threatening disease.

Of the various types of refined, concentrated sugars, none, except perhaps for molasses, has any advantage over the other. Brown sugar is table sugar with caramel color and insignificant traces of several nutrients. Turbinado sugar is simply white table sugar with a touch of molasses. Raw sugar is table sugar mixed with a small amount of beet pulp, but does not contain even a trace of appreciable fiber. Honey has only trifling quantities of a few minerals, chiefly phosphorus, potassium, and calcium. Honey's one plus is that it can be as much as 40 percent sweeter than an equivalent amount of white sugar, which means that you can use less to satisfy your sweet tooth. Molasses, the brownish liquid that remains after sucrose crystals are extracted from sugar beet or sugarcane, is probably the best of the refined sugars because it's a good source of calcium, iron, and potassium. Those darkest in color have the highest concentration of nutrients, with blackstrap molasses heading the list.

Remember that much of the sugar you consume is likely to be hidden in items you don't necessarily think of as being sweet. For example, tomato ketchup contains quite a bit of sugar; canned soups may contain as much as 3 teaspoons of sugar per serving, and sugar accounts for up to 50 percent or more of the weight of some ready-to-eat breakfast cereals. Other hidden sources of refined sugar include frozen dinners, tomato sauces, nondairy creamers, crackers, breads, bread-crumb mixes, bouillon cubes, bottled salad dressings, peanut butter, and cured meats, to name a few. (Even more important, the last three items are very high in fat.) Look at the label.

What sweetener is recommended on the Pritikin Lifetime Eating Plan? Unsweetened apple juice concentrate, sparingly used, is satisfying and is a source of some vitamins and minerals (which is why it appears in our recipes). In addition, it's very sweet, which means you don't have to use much of it to achieve a sweet flavor in your cooking.

REFINED SUGARS

Refined sugar isn't fattening because of its calories alone, but because it packs an oversupply into a very small quantity of food; that is, it has a high caloric density, meaning it can easily be overconsumed. Take, for instance, a large pear and a lollipop: Each choice contains roughly 100 calories. However, the fresh fruit also gives you vitamins, minerals, trace elements, water, and fiber, ingredients that make it both highly nutritious and naturally filling. By contrast, the lollipop supplies sugar and syrups (more sugar); its 100 calories are worth little to your health, and it is also far less satisfying than a large pear. You're likely to "overeat" foods like the lollipop long before you've curbed your appetite or filled your stomach.

EMPHASIZING UNREFINED CARBOHYDRATES

Like refined sugars, complex carbohydrates have been overrefined and overprocessed—and thereby robbed of much of their natural fiber and many of their nutrients. So it's best to eat complex carbohydrates in an unrefined or minimally refined state. Unfortunately, refined complex carbohydrates are far more likely to show up in the typical American diet than their more wholesome counterparts. What's worse, in the form of pastries, cakes, cookies, and even "enriched" white bread, these refined ingredients are also paired with harmful fats and refined sugars. In addition, refined carbohydrates, both sugars and starches, tend to trigger higher insulin levels and increased serum triglycerides (fats in the blood), which may increase the risk of heart disease.

One of the ways the body deals with an excess of rapidly absorbed sugar is to convert it into fat in the liver, which then sends it out to the fat cells in VLDL particles. The increase in VLDLs can lead to increased serum triglycerides and total cholesterol, as well as to decreased HDL cholesterol, which can create problems for those who already have heart and blood-vessel disease. By contrast, unrefined carbohydrate foods that are rich in fiber (especially soluble fiber) actually *lower* blood triglycerides in most people because they don't increase levels of insulin (which stimulates the liver to produce triglycerides) as much as refined carbohydrates do.

For all these reasons, it's best to eat unrefined carbohydrates whenever possible. At the very least, limit your refined carbohydrates, and make refined complex carbohydrates no more than 25 percent of your total complex-carbohydrate intake (which means it's okay to have an occasional piece of French bread or a plate of "white" pasta in a restaurant when there is no less refined alternative. White pasta is certainly preferable to french fries!). Remember, however, that carbohydrates stripped of their valuable fibers and nutrients will not lower cholesterol or lower the risk of colon cancer as much as their unrefined counterparts.

Recently, there have been claims that a high-carbohydrate diet will not reduce cholesterol any more effectively than a diet high in olive oil will. This is true only if a diet high in *refined* carbohydrates and low in fiber is compared to a diet high in a monounsaturated fat such as olive oil. The refined-carbohydrate, low-fiber diet and the diet high in monounsaturated fats both have the same effect on total serum cholesterol—a neutral one. And since most fats raise HDL (or "good") levels of cholesterol, and refined carbohydrates do not, the lowered ratio of total cholesterol to HDL will appear to favor olive oil over refined carbohydrates. This is worse than comparing apples and oranges! But if you get most of your carbohydrates from unrefined products rich in soluble fiber, you'll get all the benefits we've covered in this chapter—including the cholesterol-lowering ones—as well as weight loss, which a diet rich in olive oil makes difficult.

THE BEST "HEALTH" FOOD

Unrefined or minimally processed foods of vegetable origin can provide the bulk of the nutrients we need in a form that the body uses easily, so you can see why unrefined-carbohydrate-rich foods should form the highest percentage of any nutrient on the Pritikin plan: about 75 to 80 percent of the total. Focus on the "good," grown-from-the-ground carbohydrates whenever possible: They're the foods that will give you optimal vigor and energy and help to control your weight. A considerable dividend is that they taste so good—and are so satisfying as the basis of your meals. Discover the pleasure of grains and fruits and vegetables whose flavor and texture haven't been masked by chemical processing and unwholesome additives like refined oils, excessive salt, and refined sugar. Splendidly compatible with your basic body chemistry, unrefined carbohydrates can increase your chances of living a longer, healthier life. They're the fuel your body works best with—and they're also what will keep you slim, bountifully nourished, and free of debilitating illness.

PART III

The New Pritikin Diet, Exercise, and Stress-Management Program

Congratulations! You're about to unroll the blueprint for a workable program to get—and stay—healthy. You now know why the Pritikin program—consisting of a good eating plan, an effective, enjoyable approach to exercise, and a healthy perspective on creating a balanced life-style—is the best way to improve your overall health, lose unwanted body fat, and add years to your life. You're right up to the minute on matters nutritional. You're ready to roll up your sleeves and get started! So in the next nine chapters, we'll set out the Pritikin program in ways that will make clear how easy, and enjoyable, it all is.

Don't worry if the first days or weeks of getting your life onto a healthy track have their awkward moments—starting anything new takes some adjustment. But as you streamline your new shopping and cooking techniques, as you revamp your tastes so you can appreciate food that hasn't been doused with butter, salt, and/or sugar, as you carve out time for exercise and relaxation, and then actually begin to see the *benefits* of all this—greater energy, a more positive attitude, healthy weight maintenance, and a dramatic decrease in your risk of life-threatening disease—you'll experience a new contentment that comes from the knowledge that you're doing *all* you can to enhance your health.

What you need first, though, are some inside secrets to get you started and to keep you on track. Things to remember and to remind yourself of—some proven tricks of the good-health trade. It's all right here in Chapter 10—our "Formula for Success." Good luck!

CHAPTER 10

Formula for Success

What do you need to get on—and stay on—the winning path to good health? Well, the very first step you take can start you on your way. That means you're on the right path now—you're reading this book! As you follow all the food, exercise, and stress suggestions you're about to learn, you'll develop an overall outlook that will help you make these healthy principles *your* principles. Since we know where that winning attitude will lead you, let's take a closer look at where it comes from.

BELIEVE IN YOUR ABILITY TO SUCCEED

This is our first and most important suggestion. You have every reason to believe you'll succeed! Dr. Albert Bandura, a psychologist from Stanford University, has coined the term "self-efficacy" to describe the trait shared by those who believe they can succeed.[1] The stronger you are in this belief, the more effort you're likely to expend changing your unhealthy habits—the more you'll want to *persist* in the face of obstacles, and dwell on your accomplishments rather than on your failures. Be your own coach, and learn to foster your own "self-efficacy." Remember that every day you're on the Pritikin program, you're one step closer to your goals. Let that inspire you!

ADOPT A NEW WAY OF THINKING— POSITIVE THINKING!

Isn't that what so much of it all comes down to—a new way of thinking? Not that all of what we offer here will be new to you, but what the Pritikin program urges you to do is put all this information together, so you can protect yourself as much as possible from the bumpy ride life sometimes takes us on.

Making any profound change in behavior—letting go of deep-seated habits—can make your "old self" rear its familiar head, urging you back to earlier, seemingly safer (because they're more familiar) patterns. These voices will no doubt sound familiar: "Every time I go on a diet, I do something to spoil it." "I can't do *anything* right." "I was just meant to be overweight, that's all." "It will be impossible for me to give up my favorite foods."

Our old selves have fashioned blanket, across-the-board ideas about what is and isn't possible, made up of lingering parental admonitions, old wives' tales, half-baked ideas about our limitations, and a good amount of fear—fear of change, fear of failure, even fear of success.

The positive news is that this old, outdated thinking can be filtered out. You can, with great effectiveness, simply talk *back* to yourself—in effect, correct yourself—whenever you hear the old negative messages. Making positive assertions to yourself can be as simple as lifting the needle off a record and replacing it in a different groove. Here are some examples, to which you'll undoubtedly be able to add many of your own.

TALKING BACK TO YOURSELF—POSITIVELY

Let's call the old negative messages "Resistant Self-Talk," and the positive replacements for those messages—the real truth about ourselves that we can use to motivate us—"Motivational Self-Talk." When you hear a negative message, respond with a positive one!

Resistant Self-Talk	*Motivational Self-Talk*
1. It's too late to change the way I live.	1. It's never too late to grow and change. In fact, I'll start right now by being positive.
2. I have no control over my health.	2. I have control over many habits that affect my health, including the foods I eat and how I choose to keep active.
3. Eating this way is too difficult.	3. Eating this way is not such a big deal. In fact, I have a lot of delicious foods and recipes to choose from.
4. I'll never be able to enjoy my favorite foods again.	4. Life isn't all or nothing. I'll do the best I can—make one choice at a time.
5. I can never stay on a diet.	5. The Pritikin plan isn't a diet—it's a way of life I can make work for me. What I've done in the past does not have to dictate what I'll do in the future.
6. I don't like to exercise.	6. I'm choosing to exercise to feel better about myself and to improve my health—and I'm discovering I *do* like it!
7. I should always be energetic and on the go.	7. I don't have to be productive and full of energy every minute to accept myself. Different energy and productivity levels are okay.
8. I can't help the way I respond—I just can't change who I am.	8. I can learn new ways of responding to people and things if I put my mind to it.
9. My mistakes and vulnerabilities make me a failure—a loser.	9. Mistakes are opportunities to grow and learn more about life.

We suggest you personalize your "countertalks"—whatever works for *you* is what we encourage you to practice. The important thing to remember is that you *can* counter those negative messages: Simply interrupt or stop them, just as you would a record playing the wrong music, and then consciously replace them with the *right* "music." Practicing positive self-talk isn't a lot of hot air—it's essential to helping you gain control of your health and your life.

GET CLEAR ABOUT YOUR DIRECTION

It's important to be very clear and specific about what you want to accomplish, because it allows you to see more clearly what you have to do. Creating a game plan is a good idea. Set up your week ahead of time: Make appointments with yourself to shop, cook, exercise, relax—all the good things you know you need to do to get healthy— and then stick to them. It's another surefire winning tactic.

And don't wait—take action *today*! This doesn't mean "Take action without thinking" or "Never relax." (Resting at the right times is just as much "doing" as exercising at the right times.) Just realize that until you take the first concrete steps to making it a reality, your goal of getting healthy is exactly that—a goal. Get started on your new program today—don't just think about it.

LEARNING FROM YOUR MISTAKES

Try as we might, sometimes we do slip up. An offer of ice cream you can't pass up, or a piece of fried chicken. A morning when you look at your running shoes and groan "No way!" then pull the covers over your head and go back to sleep.

You might even allow a negative domino effect to take you (quite quickly!) from acknowledging you've goofed to the full conviction that you're totally lost, doomed to failure, and can never hope to get back on track again. So the ice cream becomes a three-scoop sundae, heavy on whipped cream . . . the chicken leg turns into half the bird, with fries on the side . . . the running shoes gather dust as you ignore them not only this morning but tomorrow, and the next day, and the next. Obviously, you tell yourself, you're not made of the right stuff. Maybe other people can get healthy, but you just don't have the willpower.

Nonsense!

It's certainly okay to be human. You can *always* recover from that first misstep, and you don't have to rack yourself with guilt every time you go off track. Remember, you can start your day over *anytime*. If you've had a lousy, stressful morning—you even had a bite of buttery Danish during your coffee break—by lunchtime that blue-plate special of sausages, french fries, and coleslaw can look awfully good. You've proven you're weak, haven't you? After all, you did eat that bit of Danish . . .

Here's where you can stop. Close your eyes, take a deep breath, and then look at your watch. It may say 12:30, but so what? You can start your day over anytime. So, go ahead—order your lunch. "Turkey breast on whole-wheat pita, with mustard and tomato." You're back on track!

HANDLING WEIGHT-LOSS SLOWDOWN

Most likely, if you keep to the Pritikin Lifetime Eating Plan, you'll lose excess fat and weight steadily—at exactly the right rate for you. But sometimes people find that they've hit a plateau where their scale weight just doesn't budge despite all their efforts. Why does this happen?

First of all, some setbacks and plateaus are probably inevitable, and some will turn out not to be setbacks after all; what seems like a dead halt where you can't drop those last 5 pounds may just be part of a normal metabolic process. One or more of the following factors may be the reason that your weight is staying the same, and none (but the last) is anything you can change. All are temporary, and you don't need to worry about them. In fact, each one of them presents you with an opportunity either to do something to improve or to realize it's okay to be exactly where you are.

If your weight does stay stuck for a while, however, some of the following factors may explain it:

- A change in medication: Starting or discontinuing certain drugs can interfere with weight loss. If you stop taking a diuretic, for instance, your body may retain more fluid than usual, which could easily boost your scale weight. Taking a beta-blocker drug could cause a temporary increase in your blood volume and have the same effect. You'll soon adjust, and your weight loss will continue.

- Menstruation: Women may gain several pounds of water weight several days before their period, which can easily mask a decrease in body fat.
- Starvation response: Here's the "setback" over which you *do* have some control, and, by definition, controlling it doesn't mean self-deprivation! The starvation response is the phenomenon that results from reducing your caloric intake drastically, as you might be tempted to do when you hit a plateau. Doing this may trigger a marked drop in your metabolic rate as your body takes steps to defend itself from what it "reads" as starvation. This can slow down weight loss and even cause you to regain fat when you start taking in more calories, since your body will be storing calories more readily than burning them. This is one of the reasons we tell you *not* to cut your daily intake to fewer than 1,000 calories for women and 1,200 for men, since it may ultimately boomerang.

Above all, don't be discouraged: Plateaus are actually good news because they represent new, lower "setpoints" that your body is striving to maintain after losing an appreciable amount of fat. (Your setpoint is the weight your body normally maintains if you are not aggressively trying to lose or gain weight.) After yielding to the effects of your eating plan, your body will pull back and resist further losses for a while—the classic plateau—before resuming its downward course.

You can lower your setpoint and step up your metabolic rate by adhering to all the principles of the Pritikin Lifetime Eating Plan and of the exercise program you'll put together for yourself. By reducing your intake of dietary fat, increasing aerobic activity, consuming more dietary fiber, and eating foods low in caloric density, you'll be doing all you can. After you reach your ideal weight, you'll level off for good by increasing your portion sizes of grains, vegetables, and fruits. Weight maintenance will then be largely automatic.

EMOTIONAL SETBACKS AND "SLIPS"

We'll deal with a lot of the emotional challenges you're likely to encounter in your day-to-day life in Chapter 17, when we talk about stress—and about the relaxation techniques we've found especially useful to manage stress. These techniques will be of special importance during the first three months or so that you're on the Pritikin program, because that's the time your emotional reactions are likely to be heightened, as they generally will be whenever you undergo any profound change, whether good or bad. What we don't want you to do is capsize—start a backslide from the nutrition and exercise program you've begun for yourself because you're reacting badly to something your boss said, or something your child just did!

One businessman, George D., couldn't understand why he'd regained 15 of the 30 pounds he'd originally lost on the Pritikin program—until he really thought about it. He had gone through a divorce, suffered from business reversals, and discovered that his daughter was experimenting with drugs—all within the same year! At first he berated himself for "not having handled things better." But then he began to focus on what he *had* continued to do: He was still exercising, which he knew was good for him, and some of his diet was on track—but pressures had triggered a backslide in his eating habits (he just wasn't focusing on the doughnuts he grabbed when the coffee trolley rolled by).

He began to see, though, that with only a few simple adjustments he could resume the healthy regimen he'd started—he didn't have to give the whole thing up because it was "all too much." He was renewing his commitment—as you can do at any time—but he *wasn't* starting at square one! What George also saw was that a considerable number of the difficulties he'd had to deal with were not of his making, and that the guilt that had made him so miserable and had driven him off track wasn't even appropriate! Moreover, he learned that there's no need to react to emotional setbacks with negative behavior, and he's better prepared now for the next challenge that comes along.

That's the kind of balanced approach that the right thinking can bring you. We don't promise you'll never suffer another disappointment in your life—we just urge you to make the nutritional and exercise program you're on such second nature that you won't derail when the ride gets bumpy. And by maintaining your good eating and exercise habits, you'll be able to handle life's events better— another way to stay healthy, as you'll learn in Chapter 17.

Here are a few pointers to help you overcome the slips that emotional setbacks sometimes lead to:

- *Learn to identify high-risk situations that might pose a problem for you.* This is really just preparing for the future. The events or circumstances that give rise to negative behavior are usually regular occurrences—even if, in the heat of the moment, you think you're being totally "spontaneous" and that "this has never happened to me before!" Take some time to figure out what circumstances usually prompt you to binge—holiday celebrations or reunions, new job assignments, having to cope with something difficult either at home or at work.
- *Take steps to prepare for challenging situations with positive action.* Once you've identified what usually throws you off track, be prepared with alternative courses of action: What alternatives might you choose instead of eating (or smoking or drinking or slacking off on exercise)? Be specific about these alternatives to negative behavior beforehand; don't depend on your future self to know what to do in a difficult moment. At the height of a challenging situation, it's easy to develop tunnel vision—no options seem available! Remind yourself that you can do a quick breathing exercise, fix yourself a cup of herb tea, take a walk around the block. Refer to the "Motivational Self-Talk" we gave you earlier: Pick up the needle and play a new record!
- *Learn to recover from the first slip.* Remember what we said about learning from mistakes—it's *not* the end of the world if you slip! You can always return to the Pritikin program, starting right now. See if you can learn anything from the slip itself: Can you identify what led up to it, something you never realized before? Ask for more support from family, friends, and colleagues; let them in on the goals you're trying to achieve, so that they can help you and root for you.
- *Remember that change means more than making one decision.* This may be the most important realization you can make, and it's certainly central to the Pritikin program. Good health comes as the result of the intermeshing of so many different factors—a good diet, a good exercise program, a good handle on the challenges of life—and each of these factors means making what are often small but crucial changes in what you eat and how you live (like walking rather than taking a cab or bus, or using a splash of vinegar instead of a splash of oil).

Also, healthy change will never come from addressing only one disease risk factor. To address the whole body and all of the health risks you face, you've got to make changes where fat, cholesterol, and sodium are concerned (in the proportions as well as in the sources of the foods you eat) *and* in your activity level. *There is no magical quick fix!* If there were, believe us, we'd be the first to tell you. Weight loss and good health come about permanently only when you've brought them into being slowly and steadily.

- *Reinforce positive efforts.* If you tend to be a perfectionist, you're no stranger to that insidious inner voice that tells you you're never doing quite *enough*. Learn to talk back by saying "I'm doing as much as I can to get better!" Every time you've made measurable progress, reward yourself—with a gift or a short trip or just a pat on the back.
- *Strive for balance.* In the same way that the Pritikin program addresses all the known risk factors for heart disease, cancer, and diabetes, we want you to have an all-encompassing vision of your own life and activity. Too much of any one thing will cause damage, imbalance. Consider a typical day in the life of the average overstressed, over-worked person—unfortunately, not much harmony or equilibrium there! But changing that may not be as hard as it seems. Sometimes you can restructure your day by the simplest of means: Get up a little earlier so you've got some time to organize your thoughts or to meditate (you'll learn this relaxation technique in Chapter 17); take a few minutes in the middle of the day to do some invigorating stretches; close your office door for ten minutes just to close your eyes and relax; plan ahead so you know there will be time for a leisurely, healthy meal when you get home. There are any number of options that can begin to restore the balance in your life. Remember, it's not enough just to *want* to change your behavior—you need to help yourself along. There's a lot you can do to make your surroundings more amenable, and it will probably take a lot less effort than you thought.

Winners face life with a positive attitude and know how to get back on track when they get off—that's what all these pointers are about. The trick is to become *conscious* of what you're doing to and for yourself, so you won't backslide unwittingly. And that's the reason for our next suggestion—to become aware of your progress, and to celebrate it!

TAKING STOCK AND SETTING GOALS

Pretend you're the manager of a general store. It's the end of a busy Thursday and sales have been brisk all week. You check to see how much flour you've got left, how many carrots and potatoes—are you getting low? Better order some more stationery and notebooks, too—those last three customers nearly cleared you out. What are you doing? Taking inventory, what any smart businessperson does to make sure things run smoothly. There's a good chance you do the same thing at work: You keep track of what you need, what you're about to run out of, what you've got plenty of at the moment.

So why not do the same for yourself—why not take stock of your *health* in the same way? You can start by determining how long it's been since you had a complete checkup—including a blood test that told you your cholesterol, triglyceride, and glucose levels. How much of the "good" (HDL) cholesterol do you have and how much of the "bad" (LDL)? Are you experiencing excess stress? Can you identify what's causing it? Are you tired, do you get headaches, are you irritable? Do you usually rush through meals and "grab a bite" without thinking about (or really enjoying) what you're eating? Are you sleeping well? Do you get enough exercise?

Out of all this should come a pretty clear picture, as well as an equally clear idea of what you might need to do about it! But remember, that doesn't mean that if you finally acknowledge you've got to lose 20 pounds you should agonize over the fact that you can't lose them *instantly*. Setting a goal is its own particular triumph; achieving the goal is another kind, one that always takes time, perseverance, and patience. Don't expect the impossible. Do, however, expect the possible—which may turn out, especially on the Pritikin program, to be miraculous enough!

To make things easier, we've put all our suggestions for monitoring your progress into one quick-glance chart (see Table 10-1, on pp. 133–34). On the left you'll find methods to monitor blood pressure, exercise, blood values, and weight; in the center, indications of what "on track" and "off track" mean; and finally, on the right, what to do to get back on track if you've gone off. Refer to this whenever you take your good-health inventory.

EVALUATING YOUR PROGRESS

Progress—not perfection. This is something to remember—and to remind yourself of frequently. As your goals become clear and you take the first steps to achieving them, you might want to give yourself periodic checkups to see how you're doing. These are *not*, as we can't emphasize enough, invitations to tear yourself down for not having achieved everything you want to achieve right away. They're

TABLE 10-1
SELF-MONITORING SUGGESTIONS

Monitoring Method	On Track	Off Track	Getting Back on Track
BLOOD PRESSURE Check every 3–6 months depending on history. Check once a week if on medication or have history of high blood pressure.	Resting blood pressure lower than 140/90 (ideal is no higher than 120/80).	Blood pressure over 140/90 on three successive readings.	Check diet. Check alcohol, fat, and salt (if salt sensitive). Check weight, exercise, and stress level. Change medication only with your doctor's supervision.
EXERCISE Check resting and recovery heart rate (see Chapter 16), blood pressure, distance, time, and speed. Check increases in flexibility.	Following your exercise program.	Skipping exercise. Overtraining signs: increased resting heart rate, fatigue, feeling stale, bored with exercise, injuries.	Check reasons for skipping: time, obligations, weather, type of exercise, etc. Alternate forms of exercise: Watch TV or listen to tapes while exercising; exercise with others or with your dog.

TABLE 10-1
SELF-MONITORING SUGGESTIONS (continued)

Monitoring Method	On Track	Off Track	Getting Back on Track
SERUM CHOLESTEROL AND TRIGLYCERIDES			
Have monthly lab tests until ideal, then every 3 months. Consult your doctor about a schedule of regular tests.	Cholesterol 160 mg/dl or lower. LDLs lower than 100 mg/dl. Triglycerides 150 mg/dl or lower.	Cholesterol and/or triglycerides increase 15 percent over ideal values or previous values.	Examine diet, exercise, and stress level. Repeat tests in 1–2 weeks. If still elevated, examine diet more closely.
WEIGHT			
Weigh once a week on same scale, in same clothes, at same time of day.	1–2 pounds per week weight loss or maintaining weight. Having a healthy attitude about food. Thinking about food as fuel.	Weight gain of 2 pounds per week. Clothes not fitting. Using food for nonfood purposes. Eating something "just this once" once a week or more. Skipping meals or eating infrequent meals.	Take one day at a time. Examine the difficult times of day or settings. Find one solution and try it for one week. Find other ways to meet nonfood needs. Increase exercise.

an opportunity to see what you *have* done, and if you're on track—and if you *are* on track, then celebrate! If you're a little off track, you'll be able to see clearly what to do. That's the spirit in which we offer the following checklist. It's not a quiz you pass or fail—it's just a series of reminders and questions that will enable you to see how well you're doing, and to pinpoint the areas where you may still need some work. Think about these things at the end of each day:

CHOLESTEROL AND FAT

Did I stay within my guidelines for high-protein foods like fish, lean fowl, and lean meat?
Did I stay within my guidelines for dairy products?
Did I avoid egg yolks and products with whole eggs?

SALT AND SUGAR

Did I avoid adding salt to my food, as well as food with excess sodium in it?
Did I avoid refined sugars?

LIFE-STYLE

Did I exercise today?
Did I take some time out for myself?
Did I avoid regular coffee and tea, and chocolate?
Did I avoid using tobacco?
Did I avoid excess alcohol?

ENERGY LEVEL

On a scale of 1 to 5, with 1 being low energy and 5 being high energy, what was my energy level today?

This checklist will help you steer your own course for the day coming up, as well as give you an idea of the day you've just been through. In Chapter 18 you'll learn our "S.I.M.P.L.E." approach to making your new way of life permanent. You'll want to refer to those techniques often, both in the first few weeks you're following the Pritikin program and in the months and years that follow. Remember, too, that you can return to any of our other suggestions—our stress-management techniques, or our techniques for resisting negative self-talk—anytime you want. Use these as a resource when things get tough, and when you have a moment to take stock of what you might need to "engineer your environment" a little more effectively. We want you to achieve all the success you can, and these are some of the ways you can set yourself up for it. Staying on track for a lifetime is the ultimate goal, and it's a goal you can achieve one day at a time. All you've got to do is take the first step—and you're already on the winning path.

CHAPTER 11

Go, Caution, Stop

What's a day on the Pritikin Lifetime Eating Plan like? On a typical morning, your breakfast might be hot or cold whole-grain cereal (maybe oatmeal or wheat flakes) with fresh berries and skim milk. Or if you've got a bit more time and the inclination, you might start with our recipes* for Banana French Toast or Oatmeal Pancakes topped with Hot Cinnamon Applesauce. A Sunday morning with the paper might inspire you to make Cheese Blintzes and add Fruit Syrup. For lunch, how about a quick whole-wheat pita stuffed with sprouts, cucumbers, and tomato with a splash of red wine vinegar, and then an apple—or spinach linguine with eggplant and Marinara Sauce, artichokes vinaigrette on the side, and strawberries for dessert?

Do you like Mexican food? Try a soft chicken taco with assorted vegetables and fresh salsa—either at home or at your favorite Mexican restaurant. Italian-food lovers enjoy our Cannelloni with Marinara Sauce, a favorite with kids and parents alike. If company's coming, look to such easy-to-prepare entrees as Teriyaki Chicken, seafood kabobs, roast turkey, Cranberry-Glazed Chicken Breast with Whole-Grain Stuffing, poached salmon, or elegant Red Snapper Veracruz.

And on the side? Wild rice, steamed asparagus, grilled corn, Scalloped Potatoes, and whole-grain stuffing are just a few possibilities. One favorite quick meal—even easier in the microwave—is a baked potato topped with beans in a snappy chili tomato sauce.

* Recipes for all dishes with capitalized names follow in Chapter 13.

137

Hungry between meals? Snack on Pritikin brand 7-grain rice cakes, fruit (try something a little exotic, like papaya!), a vegetable salad, a quick broccoli bisque, salsa-marinated mushrooms—maybe even just a slice of whole-grain bread with a little Pritikin brand no-sugar-added fruit spread. Desserts range from a simple dish of melon cubes to our Cheesecake recipe (with a blueberry variation) or Apple-Date Cake with hot brandy sauce. In short, there's no "typical" day on the Pritikin plan—you've got as many choices as your time, imagination, and appetite allow.

To help you make your choices, the Pritikin Lifetime Eating Plan puts all foods into one of three different groups: "Go," "Caution," and "Stop."

"GO"

As you'd expect, all foods in the "Go" category are the ones you want to eat—they're the most healthful. All of our menus are created around these most desirable foods.

Whole grains and starchy vegetables. All whole grains (for example, wheat, oats, rye, barley, corn, and brown rice) in the form of breads, cereals, pasta, rice, and crackers (prepared without oils and fats)—for example, whole-grain bread, whole-wheat spaghetti, oatmeal, rice crackers. You can also choose from among starchy vegetables such as potatoes, yams, and winter squashes. Refined grains and grain products, such as white flour, white rice, and sourdough bread, may be eaten provided they do not exceed one-quarter of total grains.

Vegetables. Fresh or frozen vegetables, as desired, raw or cooked, without added fat or salt—for example, broccoli, carrots, cauliflower, lettuce, onions, and tomatoes. Include dark green and yellow or orange vegetables daily. Vegetable juice may be substituted for up to one-quarter of vegetable servings.

Fruits. Whole fruit, fresh or frozen, is preferred; also fruit canned in its own juice, dried fruit, fruit juice, and fruit juice concentrate. (Think of "whole" as meaning "as grown"—unprocessed. For example, a whole apple is preferable to applesauce, which is preferable to apple juice. In this sense, "whole" isn't an indicator of quantity:

Whereas whole pineapple is a better choice than pineapple juice, you don't have to eat an entire pineapple!)

Legumes. Peas and beans—for example, chick-peas (garbanzos), green peas, lentils, and black, brown, pink, anasazi, and pinto beans.

Nuts. Chestnuts.

Dairy. Nonfat plain yogurt; nonfat or skim milk; nonfat cheese, such as dry-curd cottage cheese, also called hoop cheese.

Fish, shellfish, lean fowl, or lean red meat. Fish is preferred over fowl, and fowl is recommended over red meat (round or flank steak). Use skinned white meat of poultry.

Soybean products. Cooked soybeans and tofu (about 40–55 percent of tofu's calories come from fat, so go easy).

Ultra-low-fat cheese. In place of fish, poultry, meat, or soybean products.

Beverages. Water, any type of mineral water, hot grain beverages, vegetable juices, fruit juices, and selected herbal teas. (As a rule, prepackaged herbal teas that are sold in filtered bags—the kind that contain everyday spices, fruit or fruit peel, and/or ingredients like rosehips, chamomile, mint, and chicory—are your best choices, used in moderation. Be sure to avoid unknown or exotic ingredients.)

Miscellaneous. Egg whites, garlic, horseradish, sapsago cheese (a hard green skim-milk cheese flavored with the powdered leaves of a legume and shaped into cones), and gelatin (all in limited quantities).

"CAUTION"

But what if you feel stuck and need to adjust your choices? Enter category 2. "Caution" foods are not recommended, and the less you have of them the better—but if you're on a business trip or a vacation overseas and aren't faced with much choice, they won't do a great deal of harm, in limited amounts. (A big warning, though, is that if you have cardiovascular disease or other serious medical problems, you should be especially wary about "Caution" foods.)

The food groups listed here are in order of decreasing desirability in terms of your health, with the least harmful group listed first. Each of the "Caution" foods has positive and negative features which you'll want to weigh carefully—depending on your health and weight-loss goals—if you choose any one of them. Here's a roundup of "Caution" foods and their pros and cons.

Sweeteners. Blackstrap molasses, barley malt, maple syrup, honey, corn syrup, rice syrup, and all refined sugars. These contain no salt, fat, or cholesterol, which is a plus, but they are devoid of fiber and, except for molasses, are a source of nutritionally empty calories.

Water-processed decaffeinated coffee and tea contain no fat or cholesterol, but the tannins in coffee and tea interfere with iron absorption.

Aspartame is also free of fat and cholesterol, but it may enhance the desire for sweets, and its long-term safety is still being questioned.

Avocados and olives. Neither supplies cholesterol; both contain some fiber and are good providers of many vitamins and minerals—but 80 percent of each one's calories come from fat (mostly mono-unsaturated), making them both concentrated sources of calories. Moreover, olives contain too much sodium.

Unsalted nuts. Walnuts, almonds, cashews, pumpkin seeds, pecans, pistachios, sunflower seeds, filberts, sesame seeds, Brazil nuts, and peanuts have a similar good/bad profile: While they are cholesterol-free and very low in sodium, as well as offering some fiber, vitamins, and minerals, their calories also come mainly from fat (65–85 percent), mostly mono- or polyunsaturated. The exceptions are tropical nuts (such as coconut and macadamia nuts), which are in the "Stop" category because they are high in saturated fatty acids (for a full discussion of these fats, see Chapter 4). Since nuts are calorically very dense, they can undermine weight loss. And while they won't raise your serum cholesterol, eating nuts would make it very hard to maintain a 10 percent fat level in your diet.

Low-sodium soy sauce and miso. These should not be used in excess. Limit your intake of foods with more than 1 milligram of sodium per calorie.

Alcoholic beverages. Alcohol contains no fat, salt, or cholesterol, but, like pure sugar, it's nutritionally empty, high in calories, and has no fiber. When large amounts are drunk regularly, alcohol raises blood pressure; this excessive consumption is a key risk factor, along with excess weight and high intake of salt, for hypertension. Excessive use is also a risk factor for stroke, and has been implicated in certain cancers. What's more (and perhaps more obvious), alcohol may stimulate your appetite and lead to poor judgment when you're deciding what to eat (beer bellies don't just come from beer—they also come from the fatty snacks you eat when you drink beer!).

Dairy. Low-fat yogurt, low-fat milk, and low-fat cheeses are, like all dairy foods, indisputably rich sources of calcium and other minerals, but they contain cholesterol and derive up to 35 percent of their calories from (largely saturated) fat—"low-fat" is clearly a misnomer! They also offer no fiber and are a concentrated source of animal protein—all of which means they can heighten your disease risks and promote weight gain as well.

Oils high in monounsaturates. Olive oil, canola oil, avocado oil, and peanut oil contain no cholesterol, but they derive 100 percent of their calories from fat, besides lacking fiber and much nutritional value.

Oils high in polyunsaturates. Corn oil, cottonseed oil, sunflower oil, sesame oil, soybean oil, safflower oil, and walnut oil. The same applies to these, which may also promote some forms of cancer, as well as increase your requirements for vitamin E. In addition, high intakes of polyunsaturated oils decrease HDL cholesterol levels. They're associated, too, with an increased formation of gallstones and with the generation of "free radicals," which may impair the immune system and promote premature aging and possibly cancer.

Why this category is labeled "Caution" should now be self-explanatory. Limit your intake of these foods—and if you do eat them, try to choose foods from the top of the list rather than the bottom.

"STOP"

"Stop" means exactly that: When faced with foods in the "Stop" category, search for "Go" and, if necessary, "Caution" foods. Even consumed in modest quantities, "Stop" foods will raise your risk for heart and blood-vessel disease, hypertension, diabetes, and some forms of cancer, among other ills. Keep intake of these foods to an absolute minimum to avoid significantly increasing risks to your health.

Animal fats, tropical oils, and hydrogenated oils. Butter, chicken fat, cocoa butter (found in chocolate), coconut oil, hydrogenated vegetable oil, lard, margarine, mayonnaise, palm oil, and shortening.

Meats. Fatty meats, organ meats, and processed meats.

Whole dairy. Cheese, cream, cream cheese, half-and-half, ice cream, whole milk, sour cream, and whole-milk yogurt.

Nuts. Coconuts and macadamia nuts.

Salt products. Table salt, sea salt, and "lite" salt in excess. Limit your intake of foods with more than 1 milligram of sodium per calorie.

Miscellaneous. Egg yolks, fried foods, nondairy creamers, nondairy whipped toppings, saccharin, and caffeinated beverages.

Here's a tip that works for everyone on the Pritikin plan, for obvious reasons: Don't keep "Caution" or "Stop" foods in the house! If you stock your shelves and refrigerator with "Go" foods, they're the foods you'll eat and get used to eating. If you have to go out of your way to gorge on fast-food chicken, burgers, or french fries, you'll give yourself time to *recognize* what it is you're planning to do and stop while you're ahead. Willpower is a lot harder to exercise when you've got a bag of chocolate-chip cookies staring at you. A big key to setting yourself up for success is learning to create a good environment—one that will encourage you to make the best food choices you can make.

You can also look at the "Go," "Caution," and "Stop" categories as a source of inspiration to come up with substitutes. Want a baked potato with sour cream? Aha! Nonfat yogurt, your "Go" list reminds you, is a much healthier substitute (try it with chives). Some spicy salsa would taste wonderful on that potato, too. For salads, you'll see that lemon juice, unsalted Dijon mustard, unsalted tomato juice, and/or any vinegar with chopped fresh or dried herbs are terrific ways to make greens delicious *without* oil. Don't let these food categories limit you—let them challenge and inspire!

HOW THE EXCHANGE SYSTEM WORKS

Many people, when they start a new food regimen, feel more secure if they've got a very specific plan that tells them exactly what and how much to eat throughout the day. It *can* be a help to spell things out for yourself in black and white at least for the first couple of weeks you're on the Pritikin Lifetime Eating Plan. Although knowing the right proportions of the right foods will soon be second nature, it doesn't hurt to make it explicit right at the beginning; this is particularly helpful if you're primarily concerned with weight loss or if you're diabetic. To fill that need for a specific plan, we use a method called the Exchange System.

"Exchanges" are simply portions or serving sizes. All foods are placed in one of five main food groups: complex carbohydrates, vegetables, fruit, dairy, and high protein. By selecting a certain number of servings from each group, the Exchange System guarantees a nutritionally well-balanced eating plan while offering a wide range of choices. In other words, you can eat whatever you wish, and still get everything you need!

If you want to follow our faster weight-loss plan—1,000 calories a day for women and 1,200 calories a day for men (but not fewer!)—all you've got to do is use the suggested portion sizes on the menus given in Chapter 13 and choose from the recommended number of servings, or "exchanges," from each food group every day (see Table 11-1, on page 144). This will shift your emphasis away from the tyranny—and tedium—of counting calories. If you prefer or even enjoy counting calories (some people do), the Exchange System will make this easier, too, since each of the foods in a group contributes essentially the same number of calories. If you don't need to follow the 1,000- or 1,200-calorie plans, you may still find these varied menu plans helpful in providing a base upon which to build. Add extra servings of complex carbohydrates, fruit, and vegetables to suit your caloric needs and individual taste. Remember, you should never let yourself get too hungry.

But instead of counting calories, simply keep in mind how many servings or exchanges are to be eaten in a given day. Thus, women would have 4 servings of complex carbohydrates and a total of $3\frac{1}{2}$ ounces of fish, lean poultry, or lean meat. Men would do the same for protein, but would bring the plan up to 1,200 calories by adding more servings of vegetables, fruit, and complex carbohydrates. The variety is nearly endless.

Remember what we've stressed from the outset: You will almost definitely lose unwanted body fat on the Pritikin plan even if you

TABLE 11-1
MAXIMUM WEIGHT-LOSS PLANS

Food	Number of Servings*	Approximate Number of Calories per Serving
WOMEN: 1,000 CALORIES A DAY		
Dairy	2	90
Vegetables	7	25
Carbohydrates	4	80
Fruit	3	60
High protein (fish, lean poultry, lean red meat)	1 ($3\frac{1}{2}$ oz. cooked)	35–55 per oz.
MEN: 1,200 CALORIES A DAY		
Dairy	2	90
Vegetables	9	25
Carbohydrates	5	80
Fruit	4	60
High protein (fish, lean poultry, lean red meat)	1 ($3\frac{1}{2}$ oz. cooked)	35–55 per oz.

* On pages 146–55 you will find tinted boxes showing the serving sizes of the various foods in the five categories, plus a tinted box for miscellaneous foods.

don't adhere to our faster weight-loss plan. But don't go below 1,000 calories a day if you're a woman, or 1,200 calories a day if you're a man—you won't be getting adequate nutrition if you do, and you'll slow down your calorie-burning metabolic rate. Yes, you'll find that your plate will be full even on the minimum levels, but don't let that convince you that you won't lose weight: You will!

THE EXCHANGES: A LOOK AT YOUR CHOICES

Here are the food groups from which you'll make your selections. You've "met" these food groups before, but this is a more complete

Complex-Carbohydrate Exchange (80 calories)	Contains primarily complex carbohydrates with moderate amounts of essential fats and protein.
Vegetable Exchange (25 calories)	Contains carbohydrates and modest amounts of protein.
Fruit Exchange (60 calories)	Contains primarily simple carbohydrates and small amounts of protein.
Dairy Exchange (90 calories)	Contains nearly equal amounts of carbohydrates and protein.
High-Protein Exchange (35 to 55 calories)	Contains protein and small to moderate amounts of fat.
Miscellaneous Foods	Items that do not fit readily into any of the first five categories.

list, and will show you once again what a wide variety of foods you have to choose from.

Complex Carbohydrates

This plentiful category includes all whole grains, cereals, pastas, flours, breads, crackers, legumes, and starchy vegetables. Grains include (but certainly aren't limited to) wheat, oats, barley, rye, rice, millet, and cornmeal. (You'll be surprised how good hot rye cereal is—a little crunchy, with a very nutty taste—and how satisfying millet and barley are for breakfast.) There's a whole range of grains that may be unfamiliar to you that you'll soon want to try. Breads, homemade muffins, pasta, and crackers prepared without refined fats or oils (like vegetable shortening) are also in this group (while not preferable, refined grains such as white rice, white flour, and sourdough bread are also included in limited amounts).

Each complex-carbohydrate exchange (or serving)—which provides moderate amounts of essential amino acids (proteins) and fatty acids, too—is approximately 80 calories. To give you an idea of portion size, one medium baked potato, one slice of whole-grain bread, $\frac{1}{2}$ cup of cooked whole-grain pasta, and $\frac{1}{2}$ cup of cooked oatmeal each represent 1 serving or exchange. To many people, $\frac{1}{2}$ cup of anything doesn't sound like much, but because these foods are so naturally filling, you feel like you're getting (because you *are* getting) plenty.

Those following the 1,000- or 1,200-calorie plans will be interested in the recommended portions for this food group: 4 for women and 5 for men. Those at their normal weight may eat freely

COMPLEX-CARBOHYDRATE EXCHANGES

Each portion provides approximately 80 calories. This is not meant to be a complete list.

VEGETABLES

Beans, dried, cooked ...... $\frac{1}{3}$ cup
Beans, lima, fresh .... $\frac{1}{2}$ cup
Chestnuts 6
Corn, kernels .... $\frac{1}{2}$ cup
Corn on the cob .. 6 inches long
Corn, popped, no oil or salt
  added .... 3 cups
Hominy .... $\frac{1}{2}$ cup
Lentils, cooked .... $\frac{1}{3}$ cup
Parsnips .... $\frac{2}{3}$ cup (1 small)

Peas, black-eyed, split,
  cooked .... $\frac{1}{3}$ cup
Peas, fresh .... $\frac{1}{2}$ cup
Potato, white, baked ... 1 (2-inch
  diam.)
Potato, white, mashed ..... $\frac{1}{2}$ cup
Potato, sweet .... $\frac{1}{3}$ cup
Pumpkin, cooked .... $\frac{3}{4}$ cup
Squash, winter .... $\frac{3}{4}$ cup
Yams, baked .... $\frac{1}{3}$ cup

BREADS AND CRACKERS (whole-grain: wheat, rye, or sourdough)

Bagel, water .... $\frac{1}{2}$
Bread, whole-wheat, rye,
  sourdough .... 1 slice
Breadsticks .... 2 (4 inches long)
Bun, hamburger,
  whole-wheat .... $\frac{1}{2}$

Bun, hot dog, whole-wheat .... $\frac{1}{2}$
English muffin .... $\frac{1}{2}$
Matzo cracker, plain .... $\frac{3}{4}$ oz.
Pita, whole-wheat .. $\frac{1}{2}$ of a 6-inch
  pocket
Rice cakes .... $\frac{3}{4}$ oz.

from this healthy category. When it comes to interesting meal planning, the combinations are almost endless. If you chose an eggless bagel at breakfast, it would count as 2 exchanges; a large shredded-wheat biscuit or $\frac{1}{2}$ cup of cooked wheat cereal would each count as 1. For later in the day, two rice cakes, half of a six-inch whole-wheat pita pocket, one slice of whole-wheat bread, or a six-inch corn tortilla would each be 1 exchange as well. One-third cup of cooked brown rice, sweet potatoes, or cooked lentils would equal 1 serving or exchange, as would $\frac{1}{2}$ cup of kernel corn, fresh peas, lima beans, and

---

BREADS AND CRACKERS (whole-grain: wheat, rye, or sourdough) (*cont.*)

Rice crackers .... $\frac{3}{4}$ oz.
Roll, whole-wheat, rye, sour-
    dough .... 1 (2-inch diam.)

Rye crackers, no salt 4
Tortilla, corn .. 1 (6-inch diam.)

FLOURS

Arrowroot .... 2 Tbsp.
Buckwheat flour .... 3 Tbsp.
Cornmeal .... 3 Tbsp.
Cornstarch .... 2 Tbsp.
Matzo meal .... 3 Tbsp.

Potato flour .... $2\frac{1}{2}$ Tbsp.
Rice flour .... 3 Tbsp.
Rye flour, dark .... 4 Tbsp.
Whole-wheat flour ...... 3 Tbsp.

GRAINS, CEREALS, AND PASTAS

Barley, cooked .... $\frac{1}{2}$ cup
Cornmeal, dry .... $2\frac{1}{2}$ Tbsp.
Cracked wheat (bulgur),
    cooked .... $\frac{1}{2}$ cup
Flake cereal .... $\frac{1}{2}$ cup
Nugget cereal .... 3 Tbsp.
Grits, cooked .... $\frac{1}{2}$ cup
Kasha (buckwheat groats),
    cooked .... $\frac{1}{3}$ cup
Macaroni, whole-wheat,
    cooked .... $\frac{1}{2}$ cup
Noodles, rice, cooked ...... $\frac{1}{2}$ cup

Noodles, whole-wheat,
    cooked .... $\frac{1}{2}$ cup
Oatmeal, cooked .... $\frac{1}{2}$ cup
Pasta, enriched white,
    cooked .... $\frac{1}{2}$ cup
Rice, brown, cooked .... $\frac{1}{3}$ cup
Rice, wild, cooked .... $\frac{1}{2}$ cup
Rye cereal, cooked .... $\frac{1}{2}$ cup
Wheat biscuit cereal ..... 1 large
    biscuit or
        spoon-size .... $\frac{1}{2}$ cup
Steel-cut oats, cooked ...... $\frac{1}{2}$ cup

most pastas or eggless noodles—any of these would be perfect at lunch or dinner. And if you want to snack, you can enjoy 3 cups of unsalted air-popped popcorn—it's the standard portion.

If you're on the faster weight-loss version, though (for example, the 1,000-calorie plan), you will choose 4 servings from this group to keep your calorie intake at the appropriate level. (We don't recommend going below 4 servings of complex carbohydrates daily.) This means you might choose oatmeal ($\frac{1}{2}$ cup) or half a whole-wheat English muffin for breakfast, perhaps one baked potato for lunch, and, at dinner, a double serving of pasta as a side dish. Since all of these foods are in the same general category, you can substitute one for the other with little impact on the nutritional balance of your eating plan: Any combination will work.

Vegetables

Here's where you really can't overdo it (unless you eat too many vegetables and not enough other complex carbohydrates, in which case you could end up losing too much weight). From artichokes to zucchini, the choices are truly bountiful. Use vegetables lavishly and inventively in salads, broths (there are some terrific vegetable soups you can make that are so filling and hearty you won't believe how low they are in calories), simmered dishes, casseroles, and stews; in medleys with rice or pasta (that $\frac{1}{2}$ cup of whole-grain macaroni triples in size when you mix it with vegetables and your favorite sauce); or served as crudités with seasoned low-calorie dips.

Enjoy 7 servings of vegetables a day! (You may find it's hard to eat that much, but you certainly won't go hungry.) High in bulk, fiber, and good taste, vegetables aren't only nutritious—they satisfy. Portion sizes, each totaling about 25 calories, are about 1 cup for raw and $\frac{1}{2}$ cup for cooked vegetables (to allow for shrinkage).

Fruits

Fresh fruits are always good because, like vegetables, they're low in fat and high in fiber. The valuable soluble fiber in fruit releases its calories at a slow, steady rate. Let your imagination take you beyond the standard apple, orange, banana, or pear to the many exotic varieties now available, such as kiwi fruit and tamarind. Frozen and

VEGETABLE EXCHANGES

Each portion equals 1 cup of raw or $\frac{1}{2}$ cup of cooked vegetables, and provides approximately 25 calories. This is not meant to be a complete list, and some other vegetables not listed here will be found listed with the Complex-Carbohydrate Exchanges.

Artichoke, whole, base and ends of leaves (1 small)	Chilies	Mushrooms	Tomato (1 medium)
	Chinese cabbage	Okra	Tomatoes, canned in juice, unsalted
	Chives	Onions, all types	
Asparagus	Coriander (cilantro)	Parsley	
Beans, green or yellow	Cucumber	Pea pods, Chinese	Tomato juice, unsalted ($\frac{2}{3}$ cup)
Beets	Eggplant	Peppers, red and green	
Bok choy	Endive		Tomato paste, unsalted (3 Tbsp.)
Broccoli	Escarole	Pimento	
Brussels sprouts	Greens*: beet, collard, chard	Radishes	
		Romaine lettuce	Tomato sauce, unsalted
Cabbage	Jerusalem artichokes	Rhubarb*	Vegetable juice, unsalted ($\frac{2}{3}$ cup)
Carrots (1 medium)	Jicama	Rutabagas	
Cauliflower	Kale	Shallots	
Celery	Leeks	Spinach*	
Celery root	Lettuce	Sprouts, assorted	Water chestnuts (4 medium)
Cilantro	Lima beans, baby ($\frac{1}{4}$ cup)	Squash: zucchini, spaghetti, summer	
Chayote			Watercress
Chicory	Mint		

* High oxalic acid content. Not a good source of calcium.

canned fruit, prepared without sugars or syrups, are also fine choices.

There's really no limit to the amount of fruit you can eat on the Lifetime Eating Plan—although, again, on the faster weight-loss plan, women have 3 servings a day, and men 4. Each fruit exchange equals about 60 calories.

FRUIT EXCHANGES

Fresh, dried, frozen, or canned fruit, without sugar or syrup. Each portion provides approximately 60 calories.

Apple .... 1 small (2-inch diam.)
Apple juice or cider........ $\frac{1}{3}$ cup
Applesauce,
    unsweetened .... $\frac{1}{2}$ cup
Apricots, fresh .... 4 medium
Apricots, dried .... 7 halves
Banana .... $\frac{1}{2}$ medium
Berries: boysenberries,
    blackberries, raspberries,
    blueberries................ $\frac{3}{4}$ cup
Cantaloupe ..... $\frac{1}{3}$ (5-inch diam.)
Cherries .... 12 large
Cranberries, unsweetened 1
    cup
Crenshaw melon .. 2-inch wedge
Dates .... $2\frac{1}{2}$ medium
Date sugar .... 1 Tbsp.
Figs, fresh ...... 2 (2-inch diam.)
Figs, dried .... $1\frac{1}{2}$
Fruit cocktail .... $\frac{1}{2}$ cup
Fruit juice concen-
    trate .... 2 Tbsp. (1 oz.)
Grapefruit .... $\frac{1}{2}$ medium
Grapefruit juice .... $\frac{1}{2}$ cup
Grapes .... 15 small
Grape juice .... $\frac{1}{3}$ cup
Guava .... $1\frac{1}{2}$
Honeydew melon ..... $\frac{1}{8}$ medium
Kiwi .... 1 large

Kumquats 5
Lemon juice .... $\frac{1}{2}$ cup
Lime juice .... $\frac{1}{2}$ cup
Loquats 13
Mandarin oranges .... $\frac{3}{4}$ cup
Mango .... $\frac{1}{2}$ small
Nectarine ..... 1 ($1\frac{1}{2}$-inch diam.)
Orange .... 1 ($2\frac{1}{2}$-inch diam.)
Orange juice .... $\frac{1}{2}$ cup
Papaya .... 1 cup
Passionfruit 1
Passionfruit juice .... $\frac{1}{3}$ cup
Peach .... 1 ($2\frac{3}{4}$-inch diam.)
Pear .... 1 small
Persimmon, native ... 2 medium
Pineapple, fresh .... $\frac{3}{4}$ cup
Pineapple, canned without
    sugar .... $\frac{1}{3}$ cup
Pineapple juice .... $\frac{1}{2}$ cup
Plantain .... $\frac{1}{2}$ small
Plums .... 2 (2-inch diam.)
Pomegranate .... $\frac{1}{2}$
Prunes, fresh .... 2 medium
Prunes, dried 3
Prune juice .... $\frac{1}{3}$ cup
Raisins .... 2 Tbsp.
Strawberries .... $1\frac{1}{4}$ cup
Tangerine ..... 2 ($2\frac{1}{2}$-inch diam.)
Watermelon .... $1\frac{1}{4}$ cup

Dairy

No matter how many total calories you're eating, whether it's to lose or maintain weight, 2 dairy servings a day are recommended. Why? While this food group is an excellent source of calcium and vitamins D and B_{12}, it's also fairly high in animal protein, which means it may

DAIRY EXCHANGES

Each portion contains approximately 90 calories and is 1 percent fat or less by weight (15 percent of calories, or less, from fat).

Nonfat milk .... 8 oz.
Nonfat buttermilk .... 8 oz.
Nonfat yogurt .... 6 oz.
Evaporated nonfat milk ... 4 oz.

Dry-curd cottage cheese or hoop
  cheese .... 2 oz.
1% or less low-fat cottage
  cheese .... 2 oz.
Nonfat powdered milk .... $\frac{1}{3}$ cup

increase calcium excretion from the kidneys and, if you eat too much, raise your serum cholesterol level as well. Servings in this group include 8 ounces (1 cup) of nonfat milk, 6 ounces of nonfat yogurt, or 2 ounces of skim-milk cheese (for example, hoop cheese—which you can use like cream cheese—and dry-curd or rinsed cottage cheese). Each portion totals about 90 calories.

High Protein

Although some types of fish are low in fat, foods high in animal protein—fish, shellfish, poultry, and red meat—are almost always relatively high in fat, protein, and cholesterol. Do look for lean meat and lean poultry to cut fat to a minimum, but remember that this is one food group which must be carefully controlled on the Pritikin Lifetime Eating Plan. Excessive intake of these high-protein foods will raise serum cholesterol in virtually everyone.

Remember, too, that dietary cholesterol *cannot* be removed from meats simply by trimming fat away or by cooking, since cholesterol is an integral part of all muscle cell membranes, not just of the fatty layer that may surround the meat or lie between the skin and the meat. A food doesn't have to be fatty to be high in cholesterol.

To keep your daily cholesterol intake under 100 milligrams, and your dietary fat to 10 percent of your total calories, it's best to eat no more than $3\frac{1}{2}$ ounces of cooked fish, skinless poultry, or lean red meat each day, regardless of whether you're losing or maintaining your weight.

Once you begin to change your perspective on meat, poultry, and fish, you'll see they don't have to be the centerpiece of a meal. You'll discover what wonderful meal *enhancers* they can be: Added to chow mein, rice, or pasta the way so many other cultures use it, a bit of meat, chicken, or fish seems to go farther and satisfy just as much as a huge slab. Think of meat and fish as the *accents*—not the foundations—of your meals.

HIGH-PROTEIN EXCHANGES

Each portion provides approximately 35 to 55 calories per ounce. High-protein exchanges are controlled because of their fat and cholesterol content. Although soybeans and tofu do not contain any cholesterol, they are higher in fat than any other legumes; 40 to 55 percent of their calories come from fat. You may select soybeans or tofu in place of fish, fowl, or meat on the Pritikin Lifetime Eating Plan.

In the chart below, note the total fat, cholesterol, and calorie contents, as well as the percentage of calories from fat, in $3\frac{1}{2}$-ounce cooked servings of the foods. (Shrimp, which appears between the solid and dotted lines, is recommended in 2-ounce portions. Foods that appear below the dotted line are not recommended.)

Meat or Fish Source ($3\frac{1}{2}$ ounces cooked)	Fat (g)	Chol. (mg)	Calories	% Calories from Fat
Abalone	0.3	54	49	4.0
Lobster, northern	0.6	72	98	5.4
Pike	0.9	50	113	7.0
Flounder	1.0	46	129	7.0
Cod, Atlantic	0.9	55	105	7.4
Haddock	0.9	74	112	7.5
Sole	0.8	42	68	10.0
Scallops	1.4	52	112	11.0
Clams	2.0	67	148	12.0
Red Snapper, mixed species	1.7	47	128	12.1
Crab, Alaskan king	1.5	53	97	14.0
Tuna, white, water-packed	2.5	42	136	16.0
Turkey, white meat	3.2	69	157	18.0

As for calories, each ounce averages from 35 up to 55; if you want to limit your intake to less than one $3\frac{1}{2}$-ounce serving a day (advisable for people with heart disease and/or elevated serum cholesterol levels of more than 240 mg/dl), you can compensate for the decreased calories with an endless array of beans, peas, and lentils, or you can

Meat or Fish Source ($3\frac{1}{2}$ ounces cooked)	Fat (g)	Chol. (mg)	Calories	% Calories from Fat
Sea bass	2.6	53	124	19.0
Halibut	2.9	41	140	19.0
Chicken, white meat	3.6	85	165	20.0
Oysters	2.2	50	90	22.0
Mussels, blue	4.5	56	172	23.0
Trout	4.3	74	151	26.0
Beef, top round	5.4	84	184	26.0
Pork tenderloin, lean only	4.8	93	166	26.1
Swordfish	5.1	50	155	30.0
Beef, flank, lean only	7.3	90	195	34.0
Lamb, lean leg	7.0	93	184	34.0
Salmon, sockeye	11.0	87	216	46.0
Sardines, Pacific, water-packed, unsalted	12.0	81	178	61.0
Shrimp	1.1	133	99	9.8
Crayfish	1.4	178	114	10.7
Chicken, dark, without skin	9.7	93	205	43.0
T-bone steak, lean	10.4	80	214	44.0
Veal, rump and round	11.2	101	215	46.0
Turkey, dark, without skin	11.5	89	221	47.0
Pork loin, top	14.9	94	258	52.0
Beef, lean ground, broiled	17.6	101	280	57.0
Beef, chuck (pot roast), fat and lean	24.4	99	337	65.0

Source: U.S.D.A. Handbooks 8-5, 1979; 8-10, 1983; 8-13, 1986; 8-15, 1987.

eat extra fruits, vegetables, and other complex carbohydrates to keep your calorie intake up to 1,000 or 1,200.

When you do select animal protein, remember the order of desirability: Fish or shellfish comes first. Shellfish are very low in both total and saturated fat and contain no more cholesterol than other flesh foods. In moderation, they can be a safe and healthy choice in the high-protein category. For example, a $3\frac{1}{2}$-ounce serving of lobster contains about 72 milligrams of cholesterol; by comparison, $3\frac{1}{2}$ ounces of extra-lean beef such as flank steak or round contains approximately 90 milligrams.

Even better shellfish news: Lobster, crab, and most mollusks— clams, mussels, oysters, and scallops—are all relatively low in saturated fat. Their cholesterol content averages only 40 to 80 milligrams per $3\frac{1}{2}$ ounces, and so they're also acceptable choices in regular servings of $3\frac{1}{2}$ ounces of cooked, edible fish. But shrimp, which is low in saturated fat compared to even lean beef, is appropriate only in 2-ounce servings because of its higher cholesterol content—more than 130 milligrams in $3\frac{1}{2}$ ounces.

Your next choice would be white-meat chicken or turkey (without skin), and then lean beef. Beef is last on the list because its total fat content is higher than that of most fish and poultry, and it has a much higher proportion of saturated fat. To keep the percentage of fat in the beef you eat as low as possible, purchase "Select Grade" instead of "Choice" or "Prime" whenever you can. For a given grade, the leanest cut of beef is round steak, with flank steak a close second.

Serving Sizes

The following serving sizes will also be helpful, since it may be difficult to gauge the weight of some of the foods in the high-protein category, and since some foods are recommended in portions other than $3\frac{1}{2}$ ounces.

Miscellaneous Foods

These include all the "Go" foods that don't fit neatly into the categories listed above and that range in calories from about 25 to 75 per serving (although sometimes less): for instance, egg whites (try an egg-white omelet), unprocessed wheat and oat bran, gelatin, garlic, sapsago cheese. Reduced-sodium or low-sodium soy sauce (no more

SERVING SIZES

Item	Raw Weight	Serving Size	Cooked Weight (edible portion)
Chicken breast	5 oz.	1	$3\frac{1}{2}$ oz.
Clams (in shell)	36 oz.	16	$3\frac{1}{2}$ oz.
Mussels (in shell)	15 oz.	33	$3\frac{1}{2}$ oz.
Oysters (raw)	4 oz.	7	—
Scallops	4 oz.	18–20	$3\frac{1}{2}$ oz.
Shrimp, boiled, medium-size	—	9	2 oz.
Soybeans, cooked (37 calories/oz.)	—	$\frac{2}{3}$ cup	—
Tofu (21 calories/oz.)	—	6 oz.	—
Ultra-low-fat cheese (less than 34% of calories from fat; 67 calories/oz.)	—	2 oz.	—

MISCELLANEOUS FOODS

In addition to the exchanges, here are recommendations for the following food items:

Item	Quantity	Calories
Egg whites	7/week	16 each
Garlic	As desired	Negligible
Gelatin, plain	1 oz./week (4 envelopes)	95/oz.
Horseradish, prepared, no salt added	1 Tbsp./day	7/Tbsp.
Sapsago (green) cheese	1–2 Tbsp./week	20/Tbsp.
Seeds (as seasoning only)	Less than $\frac{1}{8}$ tsp./day	Negligible
Soy sauce (low-sodium)	1 tsp./day	Negligible
Teas: selected herbal	Moderate amount	Negligible
Unprocessed bran	1–3 Tbsp./day as needed	9/Tbsp.

than 1 teaspoon per day) and horseradish (1 tablespoon per day) are featured in limited amounts.

It's best to avoid whole eggs (and eat only the whites) since one yolk alone supplies more than double your daily quota of cholesterol—a whopping 213 milligrams—and about one-fifth of the calories in an egg yolk come from saturated fat.

TAKING THE PLUNGE

To help ease you through the transition (and get you started on the controlled-calorie phase of the eating plan—*if* you want to take the faster weight-loss option) the "48-Hour Gear-Up Guide" in Table 11-2 (see pages 158–59) will simplify your meal planning and food shopping for the first two days. The meals listed there will provide 1,000 calories a day. Select one food (two for vegetables) from each of the groups listed opposite each meal. If you want to increase the number of calories, just add more vegetables, fruit, or complex carbohydrates.

As you can see, the Gear-Up Guide is organized somewhat like a restaurant menu. We've intentionally kept it simple to make the transition easy—but your food choices can be much more exciting (as you'll see when you get to Chapter 13, "Menus and Recipes"). Of course, there's also no reason why you can't make it even more simple than it is—if you love spaghetti with Marinara Sauce, have it more than once a week! Mix-and-match possibilities are limited only by your own tastes and imagination.

IT COULDN'T BE EASIER

Remember, the beauty of the Pritikin Lifetime Eating Plan is its simplicity. To improve your health (and, quite possibly, your looks!), just follow the concepts you've learned and remember these two important points:

- Even if you're limiting your calories to 1,000 or 1,200 a day, you can stop counting! The Exchange System does it for you. All *you* have to do is keep track of the total number of servings you have on a given day.
- Whether you're on the regular Pritikin Lifetime Eating Plan or going for quicker weight loss, remember: no more than 2 dairy servings and no more than $3\frac{1}{2}$ ounces of high-animal-protein foods a day! That's not only for your weight, but also for your health.

MAKING THE TRANSITION

Here are some general guidelines that other followers of the Pritikin program have found helpful for getting started on the Lifetime Eating Plan.

- Eat a variety of foods from each of the food groups in the "Go" category.
- Eat three full meals a day and eat snacks between meals, choosing from fresh vegetables, fruits, whole grains, starchy vegetables, and chestnuts.
- Avoid highly salted, pickled, and smoked foods. Limit foods that have more than 1 milligram of sodium per calorie so you will not exceed an approximate goal of 1,600 milligrams of sodium per day. (Soon you won't miss the taste of salt at all, and you'll wake up to so many other flavors.)
- Flavor your food with herbs and spices instead of salt (there are terrific hints on how to do this in Table 12-1, on pp. 168–70).
- Adopt new cooking techniques to control your intake of fat and oil: broil; steam; or poach or simmer in water, broth, or wine (again, great ideas in Chapter 13).
- Plan ahead by carrying appropriate foods with you: packets of no-oil salad dressing, herb tea bags, an envelope with dry nonfat milk (look for more tips in Chapters 14 and 15).

And good health, after all, is what we're about. The Pritikin Lifetime Eating Plan is the bedrock of the Pritikin program—it guarantees health benefits you can derive from no other program, far and above weight loss. And you begin to enjoy those benefits the day you begin to "eat healthy." So let's go right into the kitchen and see just how delicious a beginning it can be!

TABLE 11-2
48-HOUR GEAR-UP GUIDE—1,000 CALORIES*

	Complex Carbohydrates (select 1 from each group)	Vegetables (select 2 from each group)	Fruit (select 1 from each group)	Dairy (select 1 from each group)	Animal Protein (select 1 from each group)
BREAKFAST	__ $\frac{1}{2}$ cup shredded wheat __ $\frac{1}{2}$ whole-wheat bagel __ $\frac{1}{2}$ cup cooked oatmeal		__ $\frac{1}{2}$ medium banana __ $\frac{1}{3}$ cantaloupe __ 2 Tbsp. raisins	__ 8 oz. nonfat milk __ 6 oz. nonfat plain yogurt __ 4 Tbsp. Mock Cream Cheese (see p. 220)	
MORNING SNACK		__ 1 medium carrot __ 4 oz. low-sodium vegetable juice __ 1 cup assorted raw vegetables			
LUNCH	__ 1 slice whole-wheat bread __ 1 6-inch whole-wheat pita	__ $\frac{1}{2}$ cup steamed vegetables with lemon and salsa __ 1 cup tossed vegetable	__ 1 medium apple __ 1$\frac{1}{4}$ cup fresh strawberries __ 1 small pear	Dairy selection from dinner may be eaten at lunch instead.	

	__$\frac{1}{2}$ cup brown rice	__ salad with no-oil dressing __$\frac{1}{2}$ cup Italian-style vegetables with Marinara Sauce (see p. 268)		

AFTERNOON SNACK	__2 low-sodium rice cakes __3 cups air-popped popcorn __1 medium baked potato	__1 cup green and red pepper strips __1 cup raw carrot and jicama __1 cup cherry tomatoes (about 6 or 7)		

DINNER	__$\frac{1}{2}$ cup whole-wheat pasta __1 medium baked potato __$\frac{1}{3}$ cup brown rice	__$\frac{1}{3}$ cup Marinara Sauce (see p. 268) __1 cup vegetable salad with no-oil dressing __1 cup steamed broccoli	__1 medium peach __$\frac{1}{2}$ cup unsweetened applesauce __15 grapes	__8 oz. nonfat milk __6 oz. nonfat plain yogurt __2 oz. hoop cheese or dry-curd cottage cheese	__$3\frac{1}{2}$ oz. broiled fish __1 baked chicken breast __$3\frac{1}{2}$ oz. sliced turkey

* To maintain weight, add more complex-carbohydrate, fruit, and vegetable servings at meals and as snacks. For 1,200 calories, select one more complex-carbohydrate, one more fruit, and two more vegetable exchanges.

CHAPTER 12

The Healthy Kitchen: A Lifetime of Good Cooking

Take a look at what's on your kitchen shelves, on the counter, in the refrigerator: What do you see? You more than likely have a range of healthy foods right at hand: pasta, rice, potatoes, lettuce, broccoli, carrots, tomatoes, oatmeal, apples . . . enough to start on the Pritikin Lifetime Eating Plan *today!*

As you learn more about what's healthy and what isn't, you'll be in for a pleasant surprise: You're *already* eating many healthy foods. As for the food that isn't—well, yes, some changes might be in order. Luckily, a lot of the "convenience" foods you like to depend on— cans of salty, fatty soup, stew, and hash—now have healthy counterparts. Making changes in the way you cook doesn't have to be traumatic!

In the past few years, many food companies (with Pritikin brand food products leading the way!) have responded to increasing consumer demand by offering healthier food; it's now possible to find a growing number of alternatives to the kind of foods that were once the supermarket norm. No longer do you have to stick solely to health-food stores—although health-food stores *are* a real boon, and if you've never shopped at one because you thought you might not recognize the food, we'll take great delight in reeducating you! And today's supermarkets have rows and rows of better choices in all the important food groups; sometimes they're shelved with the tradi-

160

tional selections, sometimes with "dietetic" or "diabetic" foods, but don't let what *they* call it confuse you. Just be alert to the wide range of choices your neighborhood market already has to offer.

MAKING IT WORK

We'll get right to the tips that followers of the Pritikin program have come up with to help them prepare healthy, good food. As with all of our suggestions, don't feel limited—let your imagination run away with you, and come up with cooking, storage, and planning ideas of your own! Here are some of ours:

Change your habits one step at a time. We're not just trying to boost your morale (important as that is) when we suggest you change your cooking—and eating—habits one step at a time. The idea is to make a transition, not an abrupt break—especially if you're afraid you can't make any changes at all! Prepare fewer high-fat, high-cholesterol, high-salt foods at the same time that you increase your intake of vegetables, fruit, whole grains, and legumes.

Cook brown rice instead of white rice, and make the chili you love with lots of peppers, mushrooms, onions, and maybe even ground flank steak. Perhaps you could change the proportions in your chicken, turkey, or tuna salad so that vegetables—and some new ones like yellow, red, and green pepper, cucumber, and radishes—predominate. Use a yogurt-herb dressing instead of mayonnaise; use lemon instead of salt. Zip up your potatoes with a spicy tomato sauce. There are so many healthful substitutions you can start to make—simple "swaps" that will make your food appetizing, delicious, and much better for you!

Try fresh fruit spreads instead of butter or margarine on whole-grain bread, and cook whole-wheat pasta instead of the refined white pasta you're probably used to. Make your own soda by pouring a little fruit juice into seltzer (or sodium-free club soda). Start using healthier versions of foods you may have thought were okay all along; on page 180 we'll give you some label-reading lessons that will teach you how to spot the hidden fat, salt, and sugar in so many of today's products. Little by little, you'll find your kitchen will appear to transform *itself* as you replace unhealthy foods with nutritious ones.

Plan your menus on a weekly basis. If you're cooking for a family, you may already plan your menus at least a couple of days in advance. The time you spend deciding what you'll cook is well invested—it makes marketing less stressful and meal preparation easier. Whether you're cooking for one or a dozen, it's no different on the Lifetime Eating Plan; in fact, menu planning is fun and easy—just look at all the suggestions we have for you!

Sit down with the recipes in Chapter 13 (and with your own imagination)—it takes only fifteen or twenty minutes each week—and create seven days' worth of appetizing, nutritious meals. Then look forward to each delicious one: salmon with Dill Sauce, lentil soup, baked apples—pasta primavera! In no time, you'll probably find you're eating better than you ever did before (you'll certainly be eating healthier). Who *wouldn't* want to follow a plan that gave them all this—and more—for a lifetime?

Cook in advance. Set a few hours aside every so often (once a week is ideal) to prepare certain items in bulk. Then refrigerate or freeze them to have on hand during the days or weeks ahead. (You might also consider getting your spouse, your kids, or a friend to give you a hand. Cooking together can be a very pleasurable experience, and it will help to demystify the Pritikin plan for everyone else.) For example, you might soak a variety of your favorite cholesterol-lowering dried beans the night before, then cook and freeze them separately in the appropriate portion size, with an eye toward the salads, soups, and stews they'll make in the week ahead. Or make a large pot of chili from which you'll eat some and freeze the remainder. Plastic containers and plastic self-sealing bags designed for freezer use make terrific storage containers.

Cook grains in generous quantities; they keep well in the refrigerator for several days and can be added to an enormous variety of dishes to extend them. (They can also be frozen in smaller, ready-to-eat portions.) We'll entice you a bit later with a complete rundown of grains that may be new to you, but for now take note that bulgur (cracked wheat) and the satisfying and intriguing quinoa (available in health-food stores and many supermarkets) are quick-cooking grains that are ready in fifteen to twenty minutes. Some grains, like brown rice, do take longer to cook, but if you prepare them in advance and then reheat them in the microwave (try adding vegetables or spices for extra flavor), they will be just about perfect. Try cooking grains in defatted, low-sodium chicken or beef stock for extra flavor. Let them stand ten minutes after cooking, then fluff with a fork before serving (or remove the lid about five to ten minutes before they're done to separate the grains).

There are wonderful Pritikin brand spaghetti sauces for pasta and other dishes, but if your market doesn't carry them yet or if you like to prepare your own, make enough to last for a week or longer and store it in large tightly capped jars or in plastic containers. (Spaghetti sauce also freezes beautifully.) Bake or steam several potatoes (or microwave them) to have on hand; if refrigerated, they will remain fresh for up to four days. Preslice some crispy vegetables such as carrots, broccoli, cauliflower, or celery and refrigerate them in water in a covered container to keep them crisp. After you've used up the vegetables, add the water to a soup stock along with any leftover rice, potatoes, beans, and vegetables you have. Add defatted stock or unsalted tomato sauce and you can enjoy one of the best soups you've ever had.

Muffins are another easy item to prepare in bulk and freeze, and there's nothing homier or more satisfying with a hot cup of herb tea as an afternoon snack. Try the recipe in this book (Oat-Bran Muffins, see p. 220) or use the low-sodium, low-fat muffin mix products you'll find in health-food stores or at your supermarket.

Balance your menus by thinking ahead. If you plan a turkey sandwich for lunch on Monday, plan a meatless dinner—perhaps Black-Bean Soup or Cheese Blintzes (see pp. 243 and 213). If you eat out regularly or know that a couple of upcoming evenings will be spent out on the town with business associates or friends, figure those meals into your plan and decide what you'll eat ahead of time.

Rely on variety and imagination. Have fun with your food planning! Breakfast can mean so much more than cereal; try fruit salad and a bagel, or an egg-white omelet with mushrooms. But if you do love cereal, try a variety. Oatmeal, millet, or brown rice makes a great breakfast cereal with bananas, cinnamon, and raisins. They make good side dishes, too—such as spicy Spanish rice with green onions, tomatoes, chili, and cumin. Or create a terrific cold salad with chopped vegetables, fresh herbs, and a little mustard or vinegar dressing. The more familiar you become with meals centering on beans, grains, vegetables, and fruits, the more your imagination will take over—and soon you'll be giving *us* lessons.

Shift the spotlight of your evening meals away from fish, poultry, or meat. Making meat the focus of our meals is simply habit—an unhealthy one. But there are so many inventive ways to use fish, chicken, turkey, or lean red meat to enhance or liven up vegetable dishes or soups made with a variety of grains or legumes. For example, put *small* amounts of meat or poultry in stir-"fries," but use plenty of vegetables; serve over rice, as in Chinese or Indian cuisine. Or make the high-fat, high-cholesterol protein foods just a small part of hearty stews and chowders rich in complex carbohydrates.

And defatted meat stocks are terrific: Since cholesterol, as you learned in Chapter 5, is only present in *animal tissues and fats,* you can use as much as you want of these defatted stocks to give all-vegetable dishes a hearty, meaty taste. Make your own stock (be sure to skim off all the fat before you cook with it), or save yourself the trouble and buy Pritikin brand canned stock. You can even use stock to "sauté" meat or vegetables, as you'll see in the recipe section in Chapter 13; you don't need fat. Using $\frac{1}{4}$ cup of liquid for every cup of cut vegetables, boil the liquid alone first, then switch to a medium flame and add the vegetables, stir-"frying" until tender-crisp. You can steam with stock, too; bring it to a full boil under the steamer basket, then add the vegetables and cook, covered, for just a few minutes. The liquid, enriched by the vegetables, can become the basis of a full-bodied sauce or soup on another day. Stock stores well in a jar or plastic container and can certainly be frozen—try freezing it in an ice cube tray so you'll have small amounts ready for "sautéing."

Try new vegetables. To your basic supply of vegetables— tomatoes, lettuce, celery, carrots, cucumbers, onions, peppers, and mushrooms—add a few exotic varieties. Take a few risks! Do jicama, Jerusalem artichoke, daikon (a radish), white turnip, arugula, radicchio, and Belgian endive sound like adventurous eating? They're actually wonderful! You'll be surprised at how much is available, and how much of it you'll love—but you have to try it first. Use your food processor or blender, according to the manufacturer's instructions, to chop or shred vegetables when you're short on time. A pressure cooker can also help by speeding up cooking time: The hardest root vegetables take only ten minutes in a pressure cooker. Even garbanzo beans (chick-peas), which normally have to be presoaked for hours before cooking, can be done in forty-five minutes in a pressure cooker. (Do be careful to follow the manufacturer's directions for cooking legumes in a pressure cooker; some sp[...] and therefore should *not* be cooked this way.)

Some canned vegetables are great to have on h[...] additions to any recipe: water chestnuts, straw m[...] choke hearts, green chilies, pimentos, and hearts o[...] ̣ust be sure to rinse them before you use them, since they may have been canned with salt.) Keep these on your pantry shelf along with the green or wax beans, beets, and (low-sodium) canned tomatoes in any form, including sauces, purees, and paste. Look for canned beans without added salt or sweeteners (canned baked beans often contain sugars or syrups), and stock up on them when you find them—they can be a quick filler in many dishes. If you have a hard time finding low-sodium canned beans, however, you can rinse regular canned beans in a colander or strainer under lots of running water to wash away some of the excess salt—a compromise, but they'll be much better for you than if you didn't rinse them at all.

SWITCHING FROM HIGH FAT TO LOW FAT

One of the most healthful changes you'll be making in your diet is removing fat and cholesterol from it. Believe it or not, it's also one of the easiest! Here are some substitutes that will automatically reduce the amount of fat and cholesterol you consume; they're an ingenious, convenient, welcome group, so consult this list often.

High-Fat Item	*Low-Fat Substitute*
Mayonnaise, sour cream	Use nonfat yogurt mixed with a small amount of nonfat buttermilk or powdered nonfat milk. Or try the Mock Sour Cream recipe on page 268. Use with fish, chicken, baked potatoes, pasta, shredded cabbage (for coleslaw), or fruit, seasoning appropriately for the dish. It's a great sandwich spread, too: Add finely chopped vegetables or fresh herbs like dill, parsley, dry or

High-Fat Item (cont.)	Low-Fat Substitute (cont.)
	prepared mustard, chives, or scallions, alone or in combination, for extra flavor. Also for sandwiches, use mustard or make your own nonfat Yogurt Cheese (see p. 264).
1 whole egg	2 egg whites (avoid egg substitutes since these contain colorings and additives, among other artificial ingredients).
Cream, half-and-half	Evaporated skim milk (or powdered nonfat milk) adds a creamy texture to sauces and soups.
Fatty meats	Round or flank steak; white-meat chicken or turkey (skinless); seafood.
Oil and fat in cooking	Wine; defatted low-sodium chicken or beef broth (or use Pritikin brand product); vinegar, lemon juice, or water; nonstick cookware. No-stick sprays do contain some oil and would be your second-best choice, though they aren't ideal.
Butter, margarine	Apple butter, no-added-sugar fruit spreads and jams, fresh fruit puree.

BECOME A PRO WITH HERBS AND SPICES

Not only will your healthy guidelines and the terrific recipes in Chapter 13 get you thinking in new directions, you'll also want to do lots of innovative cooking on your own. One of the easiest and most effective ways to make your meals deliciously inviting is to use herbs and spices. Plus, it's fun! With these seasonings (some of which, by the way, make great alternatives to salt in many foods) you can brighten up or give wonderful new flavor to almost any dish, from appetizers to desserts. You can add international flair, or just a touch of sophistication—whatever you'd like. Here's a crash course in using them.

As a general rule, "a spice is hot, an herb is not." Thus, most spices (for example, cloves, ginger, sage, cinnamon, mustard, and cardamom) are strongly aromatic, lending a pronounced "nip" or "bite" to foods, whereas herbs (like basil, chives, tarragon, and dill) usually contribute more subtle flavors. (There are, however, exceptions in both cases.)

When cooking with herbs and spices, remember that they're best used to enhance or complement the natural flavors of foods, not to overpower or mask them, as salt so often does. Since a little goes a long way, use a bit of restraint when experimenting with an herb or spice for the first time. Of course, there are no "right" herbs or spices for a particular food, nor are there any "right" amounts to use—your own taste is the ultimate guide. Whatever your preference, though, you'll probably find our herb and spice chart a good guide for flavoring ideas (see Table 12-1, on pp. 168–70).

To preserve both taste and aroma, store all dried herbs and spices (commercial or home-dried) in airtight jars or nonporous containers in a cool, dark, and dry place. Never store them near the heat and moisture of a stove, and do keep them away from direct sunlight, which bleaches color and reduces strength. Be sure, however, to keep your herbs handy, within easy reach of your food-preparation area, so it will be easy to use them regularly.

Dried herbs and spices are best if used within six months to a year, so you might want to write the date you bought herbs and spices (or stored homemade) on the containers. On the other hand, some people just judge them by aroma and taste: If you have to sniff when you open the container, or use a lot to get the flavor you want, chances are the seasoning has lost most of its punch.

If you're just beginning to use herbs and spices, you'll find the following suggestions for cooking with these *real* flavor enhancers helpful:

- To maximize the flavor of dried herbs, soak them for several minutes in a liquid to be used in the recipe, like stock, lemon juice, or vinegar.

TABLE 12-1
COOKING WITH HERBS AND SPICES

Seasonings for Vegetables

Asparagus	Mustard seed or tarragon
Lima beans	Marjoram, oregano, sage, savory, tarragon, or thyme
Snap beans	Basil, dill, marjoram, mint, mustard seed, oregano, savory, tarragon, or thyme
Beets	Allspice, bay leaves, caraway seed, cloves, dill, ginger, mustard seed, savory, or tarragon
Broccoli	Caraway seed, dill, mustard seed, or tarragon
Brussels sprouts	Basil, caraway seed, dill, mustard seed, nutmeg, savory, or tarragon
Carrots	Allspice, bay leaves, caraway seed, dill, fennel, ginger, mace, marjoram, mint, nutmeg, or thyme
Cauliflower	Caraway seed, dill, mace, or tarragon
Cucumbers	Basil, dill, mint, or tarragon
Eggplant	Marjoram or oregano
Onions	Caraway seed, mustard seed, nutmeg, oregano, sage, or thyme
Peas	Basil, dill, marjoram, mint, oregano, poppy seed, rosemary, sage, or savory
Potatoes	Basil, bay leaves, caraway seed, celery seed, chives, dill, mustard seed, oregano, poppy seed, or thyme
Spinach	Basil, mace, marjoram, nutmeg, or oregano
Squash	Allspice, basil, cinnamon, cloves, fennel, ginger, mustard seed, nutmeg, or rosemary
Sweet potatoes	Allspice, cardamom, cinnamon, cloves, or nutmeg
Tomatoes	Basil, bay leaves, celery seed, oregano, sage, tarragon, or thyme
Green salads	Basil, chives, dill, or tarragon

Seasonings for High-Protein Foods

Fish	Basil, bay leaves, dill, fennel, marjoram, parsley, rosemary, tarragon, or thyme
Meat	Bay leaves, fennel, marjoram, oregano, parsley, rosemary, tarragon, or thyme
Poultry	Chervil, marjoram, parsley, rosemary, sage, savory, tarragon, or thyme

TABLE 12-1 (continued)
COOKING WITH HERBS AND SPICES

Seasonings that add a "salty" flavor
Celery seed or powder
Garlic, fresh or powdered
Onion flakes or powder
Parsley
Soy sauce ("lite" style)
Fresh lemon juice and peel bring out
   the natural saltiness in foods.
Hot spices may satisfy your desire for
   a salty taste; try chili spices,
   red pepper sauce, or cayenne.

For a "sweet" flavor
Allspice, cardamom, cinnamon,
   clove, ginger, mace, mint,
   nutmeg, or vanilla

For a "licorice" flavor
Anise seed, fennel, star anise, or
   tarragon

For an "ethnic" flavor
Use the following singularly or in combination:

Chinese	Cayenne, cilantro, curry, fennel, garlic, ginger, hot mustard, or star anise
French	Chervil, nutmeg, or tarragon
German or Scandinavian	Caraway, cardamom, cinnamon, dill, garlic, lemon, or paprika
Indian curries	Cinnamon, coriander, cumin, fenugreek, garlic, saffron, or turmeric (see recipe, page 170)
Italian	Fennel, garlic, marjoram, oregano, parsley, rosemary, or sweet basil
Mexican or Latin American	Chili-pepper flakes, chili powder, cilantro, cumin, or oregano
Middle European	Sweet marjoram

For a "poultry" flavor
Bay leaves, marjoram, parsley, rosemary, sage, or thyme
Grains and legumes can be flavored by cooking them in a stock
   seasoned with these herbs.

Herb blends

For tomatoes	1 part savory, 4 parts basil, marjoram, parsley, and thyme combined

TABLE 12-1 (continued)
COOKING WITH HERBS AND SPICES

For salads	4 parts basil, celery seed, chervil, chives, marjoram, parsley, and tarragon combined, 1 part savory and thyme combined

Bouquet garni
1 bay leaf
$\frac{1}{4}$ tsp. crushed
   red pepper
3 or 4 sprigs
   parsley
$\frac{1}{2}$ tsp. dried
   thyme

Curry powder

$\frac{1}{2}$ Tbsp. cardamom	$1\frac{1}{2}$ Tbsp. cumin seed
$\frac{1}{8}$ tsp. cayenne	1 Tbsp. fenugreek
$\frac{1}{2}$ Tbsp. cloves	$1\frac{1}{2}$ tsp. turmeric
6 Tbsp. coriander	

(You wouldn't need to do this, however, for a long-simmering soup or stew.)
- Add herbs during the last thirty to forty-five minutes of cooking—they lose their flavor with prolonged exposure to heat.
- For cold foods seasoned with herbs and spices, flavor develops with refrigeration time. So chill the dish several hours or overnight for best flavor.
- For foods served hot, add whole spices early. Add ground spices, which release their flavors more quickly, near the end.
- Use frozen herbs in the same amounts as fresh. Add them in their frozen form to foods that are heated; allow them to thaw before adding to foods served cold.

ANIMAL PROTEIN—THE HEALTHY WAY

Choose seafood, lean poultry (not duck and goose, which are too high in fat), and lean beef (round and flank cuts) in that order of preference; avoid organ meats and processed meats like bacon, sausage, and hot dogs. While some fish, such as mackerel and salmon, can be high in fat, they are also rich in beneficial omega-3 fatty acids (as long as they are harvested in their natural cold-water habitat), which are associated with a reduced risk of coronary heart disease (see Chapter 4 for more information on omega-3)—so they can be one of your once-daily $3\frac{1}{2}$-ounce high-protein portions. However, since shrimp is somewhat higher in cholesterol than are other seafoods, it's best to keep portions of shrimp closer to 2 ounces instead of $3\frac{1}{2}$. (With all this talk of ounces, you may want to consider buying an inexpensive food scale to help you determine your portion sizes, although after a while you'll be able to gauge portions by eye. As a general rule—but beware if you've got big hands!—a $3\frac{1}{2}$-ounce portion of cooked meat or fish will cover the palm of your hand.)

Scallops, oysters, mussels, crab, lobster, and clams are somewhat lower in cholesterol and can be eaten in $3\frac{1}{2}$-ounce portions. If you like canned fish, choose the water-packed variety without added salt. Fortunately, neither cooking nor canning significantly affects the level of omega-3 fatty acids.

Some popular producers of chicken and turkey are now marketing birds with up to 25 percent less fat. Read labels to make the best choices. Avoid pre-basted turkeys since they are injected with saturated or partially hydrogenated oils (which raise cholesterol levels), may also be high in salt, and contain sugar, artificial colorings, and sodium-based compounds. Buy meat in "Select Grade," if available, since it is lower in fat than "Choice" or "Prime." (In response to consumer pressure, beef producers are now striving to breed cattle with minimal fat, so keep your eyes open for "ultra-trim," "extra lean," and other such meats from animals specially bred for leanness.)

But aren't the leanest meats less tasty and less tender than their fattier counterparts? Not if you take the right care in cooking them. Methods like braising, roasting, and pressure-cooking (see p. 185) preserve flavor and keep meats moist. Cook with broth, tomato sauce, or wine along with herbs and vegetables like onions, mushrooms, peppers, fresh parsley, and garlic. Meats yield up their own liquids, so added juices or fats (except for a little water) are rarely needed. Do skim off any fat that rises to the surface, however.

While they're expensive, game meats such as rabbit and venison are lower in fat than beef, pork, and lamb and are also relatively free of chemical residues and growth-stimulating hormones. Buffalo (bison), bred without chemical additives, is even lower in fat than lean beef. Fresh lean game and a wine marinade make a perfect "marriage of flavors"—and the beginnings of a very special meal. Try it!

DAIRY

Nonfat dairy products are preferred because most others contain cholesterol and saturated fat, and thus contribute to cardiovascular disease. Even products labeled "low-fat" (such as 2 percent low-fat milk, which is 2 percent fat by weight) can derive 35 percent of their calories from fat. Skim milk, uncreamed cottage or hoop cheese, nonfat yogurt, and nonfat dry milk are all great substitutes for whole-milk dairy foods and can be the basis for delicious recipes. For cooking or baking, you may prefer evaporated skim milk since it has a thicker consistency than nonfat milk. But it's also proportionately higher in calories, so it should be used sparingly. Sapsago, a sharp, pungent, nonfat green cheese, can be grated to flavor foods, instead of Parmesan. Since sapsago is high in sodium, though, use it very judiciously—no more than 2 ounces a week.

CHOICE CHEESES

Ultra-low-fat cheeses may be eaten in moderation (portion size is 2 ounces), as long as they are low-sodium and derive no more than 34 percent of their calories from fat. (You'll find a formula for calculating the percentage of fat in a food in the box on pages 180–81. Use it to "pretest" foods you may be unsure about.) These cheeses are especially good melted. Top a slice of multi-grain bread with 1 ounce of ultra-low-fat cheese, plus some chopped raw vegetables (onions, mushrooms, peppers) and spices (basil or oregano, perhaps), and broil for a savory grilled cheese treat. Remember that to keep your cholesterol levels safe, these cheeses are to be used in place of—*not* in addition to—your daily portion of fish, fowl, or meat, and that the portion size is 2 ounces rather than $3\frac{1}{2}$.

GRAINS—AND MORE GRAINS

Variety, in this category, is an understatement. There is *such* an abundance of grains, and new and exotic varieties keep appearing, not only in health-food stores, but in supermarkets as well. Brown rice, brown basmati rice, wild rice, wehani (a California whole-grain rice), barley, millet, cracked wheat (bulgur), oats, rye, whole-ground cornmeal, wheat berries, triticale (a cross between wheat and rye), pastas made from whole grains or Jerusalem artichoke flour, soba and other Oriental noodles, and the more exotic grains like amaranth and quinoa—you've got endless possibilities for casseroles, salads, main dishes, side dishes, and cereals.

It's true that grains are easier to find than nutritious bread: Most supermarket breads contain small amounts of saturated or hydrogenated fats, and are baked with refined flours, dough conditioners, sugar, excessive sodium, and other additives. (Whole-wheat pita bread is always a good choice, though, and is perfect for sandwiches and dips.) Pritikin brand breads, as you'd expect, are made from whole grains, without fat, and they're appearing in more and more supermarkets and health-food stores across the country.

And here's where you can rely on your health-food store to really help out. They frequently offer a number of interesting multi-grain and sprouted whole-grain breads made without undesirable ingredients. These recipes may be a mixture of oats, corn, rye, cracked wheat, brown rice, millet, barley, and even lentils; like other loaves, they store easily in the freezer. These are satisfying, flavorful breads—again, you won't feel deprived of the sugar and fat. The taste of whole grains is so much better without all that doctoring!

Avoid most commercial brands of crackers: Instead choose Scandinavian flatbreads, unsalted rye crackers, crispbread, whole-wheat matzo, rice cakes, unsalted whole-grain or sourdough pretzels (some pretzels are free of oils and shortening).

Cereals from the big name brands now offer hope: The list of fiber-rich ready-to-eat cereals that contain little or no refined sugar has grown substantially in the past several years, and shows little sign of stopping. Look for flakes, puffs, "crispies," and other varieties made from whole or mixed grains, including brown rice, oats, corn, millet, barley, rye, wheat, and amaranth. Many of these (like amaranth flakes) are still more common in health-food stores, but you'll find many others—traditional favorites such as shredded wheat (or shredded wheat and bran) and raisin bran, as well as lots of interesting new varieties, many bearing familiar brand names—right on the supermarket shelf.

Be careful about other cereals; read the labels. Many contain a lot of salt, refined sugar, and tropical and/or hydrogenated oils ("natural" does not necessarily mean healthful—beware of misleading advertising ploys). Some cereals are made with several different sweeteners, which you'll find scattered throughout the list of ingredients (see "Label Logic," p. 180); they are easily missed, so watch out for them. Look for words with the suffix "-ose" (for example, dextrose, fructose, maltose)—a tip-off to added sugar. While small amounts of added sugar aren't a big concern, if a cereal to which you haven't even added fruit tastes overly sweet, it probably contains an excessive amount of refined sugar.

One cereal that you can easily make is Granola (check out the recipe on p. 215!). It stores wonderfully, and can be eaten as a snack as well as a cereal.

As for hot cereals, always pick the ones with unrefined grains—they're the best sources of B vitamins, minerals, and fiber, as well as protein. Here's a rundown of grains for hot cereals:

Wheat. Whether this grain is rolled, flaked, cracked, or ground (either coarse or fine), all versions that preserve the bran and germ and add no other ingredients have roughly the same nutritional value. Look for the words "whole wheat" and "whole grain"; avoid farina, from which the bran and often the germ have been removed. While it's best to choose no more than 25 percent of your complex carbohydrates from refined grains, be aware that products labeled "enriched" add back some (but never all) of the original ingredients lost in the refining process. Since they are rarely returned to their natural ratio, limit such "enriched" refined grains to 25 percent or less. (Note that sourdough, French, and Italian breads, unless they've been made with whole grains, also fall into this category.)

Oats. Oats seem to be especially "trendy" right now—which is good news! Major brands offer nutritious oat cereals and other products, so keep on the lookout for them. When oats are milled, their bran and germ are left intact; only the inedible outer hull is removed. What remains is the groat, from which a number of delicious healthful variations are formed, including:

Old-fashioned or rolled oats: The groats are sliced, slightly steamed, then rolled into flakes and dried. The advantage is good nutrition in short order (they take only five minutes to cook).

Steel-cut oats: The groats are simply cracked. You cook them for as little as ten to fifteen minutes, and the result is a tasty porridge. These are available in health-food stores and often in the health-food sections of supermarkets.

Oat bran: This part of the oat grain is a good source of soluble fiber and has been getting a lot of publicity recently as a cholesterol reducer—which it is when it's part of an eating plan that's low in saturated fat and cholesterol.

Rye. Whole-rye cereal has a crunchy, nutty texture and, along with "cream of rye" (a smoother, more delicate cereal), can be found in health-food stores. It's a nice change.

Corn. Cornmeal makes an excellent smooth, creamy cereal. Look for the words "unbolted," "stone-ground," or "whole grain" on the package. Both yellow and white cornmeal can contain the germ and high-fiber bran (but if the box says "degerminated," it means it's been refined and is less preferable).

Rice. Rice isn't only a terrific staple for lunches and dinners—brown-rice "cream" (a hot cereal available in health-food stores) brings the benefits of rice to breakfast, too; it's a quick-cooking, nutritious cereal. And regular brown rice with bananas, cinnamon, and some nonfat milk makes a hearty morning meal as well.

Barley and millet, as well as other, perhaps unfamiliar, grains we've already mentioned (triticale and quinoa, for example), also make excellent hot breakfast cereals, as does kasha (buckwheat groats). Remember that grains cooked earlier in the week are as good for breakfast as they are for dinner (they reheat beautifully in the microwave), served hot or cold with skim milk, raisins, berries, or other fruit, and a sprinkle of cinnamon.

And, of course, in addition to all these grains, there are probably more good packaged hot cereals readily available at your neighborhood market than you ever thought possible. Those with combinations of four, five, or even seven grains are particularly interesting, and offer good variety.

SAUCES, STOCKS, AND SALAD DRESSINGS

This category is full of surprises—and secrets to transforming foods you may feel are too bland into great-tasting dishes. You may have thought you couldn't possibly do without oil, butter, or cream in certain sauces and dressings, so be prepared to learn how wrong you were!

First of all, nonfat milk can replace cream or whole milk in white sauces for meats, vegetables, pasta, or other grains—and will yield a lighter flavor. Mix 2 tablespoons of unbleached flour with each cup of nonfat milk, add fresh and dried seasonings, then heat and stir until thickened. Or you can add cornstarch (usually 1 tablespoon to 1 cup of milk) for the same results. Take the leftover liquid from cooking meats, poultry, or fish (chilled and skimmed of its congealed fat) and, depending on how much liquid you have, add nonfat milk, nonfat dry milk, or canned evaporated skim milk (diluted if necessary) for richness. Thicken as suggested above and season to taste: You've now got an elegant sauce. You can also thicken a sauce simply by reducing it: Boil it until some of its liquid has evaporated. To thin a sauce simply add water, broth, or nonfat milk.

It's easy to make your own chicken stock with any chicken parts (even backs and necks) and assorted vegetables, including carrots, celery, onions, bay leaf, parsley, and garlic. Cover with water, bring to a boil, lower heat, then simmer, covered, for 2 to $2\frac{1}{2}$ hours. Strain and cool, then spoon off from the surface and discard any accumulated fat. Seasonings can change at your whim—there's no one official way to make chicken soup, as you'll find out by querying people at random! (Or you can simply buy Pritikin brand canned chicken or beef stock—we've already gone to the trouble for you.)

You can make a vegetable stock simply by omitting the poultry and adding some unsalted canned tomatoes for more flavor, color, and richness if you wish. Or puree some cooked vegetables like carrots or broccoli and add them instead, for color, body, and flavor. Stock can be frozen either in plastic seal-top containers or, as we mentioned a bit earlier, in ice cube trays (remember that you can use stock to "sauté" other foods and that one or two cubes of stock will cover a medium-size skillet nicely). Anything you can cook in boiling water, you can cook in stock—remember that when you want a more strongly flavored rice or other grain.

As for salad dressings: What, no oil? Participants at our Pritikin Centers can choose from a range of wonderful oil-free dressings—from creamy to vinaigrette—and now they're available in many supermarkets as well. These bottled dressings are also free of all the fats, excess sodium, and sugar you'll find in most other commercial brands (even those labeled "lite" or "reduced-calorie").

Try our Mock Sour Cream recipe on page 268; it can form the basis of the most satisfying creamy salad dressings. Mix it with chopped herbs, or some mustard (add a bit of curry—it works especially well in a mustard dressing), or finely diced raw vegetables and perhaps a bit of unsalted tomato juice or tomato sauce—again, the possibilities are endless. And don't limit yourself to greens. You can use Pritikin brand bottled dressings or those you prepare yourself as marinades and in pasta salads, too.

Salads don't have to be only lettuce, tomato, and cucumber, either: Make them hearty by adding beans or sprouts, cooked bulgur, rice or barley, or homemade croutons. For a simpler, lighter finish to your salad, consider rinsed capers, grated sapsago cheese, balsamic vinegar or any of the numerous other "gourmet" vinegars on the market (like raspberry or other herbed vinegars), unsalted tomato juice, or even a leftover cold soup like gazpacho, which can make a terrific dressing. Pimentos, horseradish, and salsa are also great salad complements. Just don't resort to high-calorie dressings! Three tablespoons of a traditional oil-and-vinegar mix could add as many as 200 calories to your salad—and pretty soon you'd be eating something almost as fatty and caloric as a hamburger!

FRUITS

Fresh and seasonal fruit should always be your primary choice, and, as we've suggested before, use your imagination: Try something a little more exotic, like papaya, kiwi, or tamarind. Fiber-rich fruit can satisfy as a snack on its own—or be sliced onto cereals, pureed into spreads or toppings, or made part of sauces or glazes for entrees. Blend fruit into shakes, or bake it into wonderful desserts. And you were afraid you couldn't enjoy anything sweet!

If fresh fruit isn't available, look for unsweetened frozen fruits, which are just as good nutritionally. Your next choice would be canned fruit packed only in water or in its own juices. Look how easy it is to turn nonfat yogurt into something even better-tasting than the oversugared commercial fruit yogurts: Just toss in some fruit!

SANDWICHES AND SNACKS

Again, the possibilities are limited only by your imagination. Here are some ideas to inspire you:

Mash any leftover spiced, cooked beans, spoon them into steamed or baked-crisp corn tortillas, top with salsa, fresh vegetables, and herbs, and you've got a great-tasting taco or tostada. Or combine the beans with nonfat plain yogurt, tomato sauce, and fresh or dried seasonings for a savory spread on whole-grain crackers or pita bread. (Every time we serve this bean dip at parties it's the first bowl to be emptied.)

Use a hearty sprouted mixed-grain bread or an oil-free sourdough to concoct a colorful vegetable "submarine" with tomatoes, chopped bell peppers, zucchini, shredded cabbage, and carrots topped with mustard, a Pritikin brand salad dressing, scallions, sprouts, and even some grated sapsago or hoop cheese. You can also make a wonderfully satisfying, healthy sandwich with a scoop of Tuna Salad or Salmon Pâté (see pp. 251 and 234). A more exotic dressing for sandwiches can be made with plain nonfat yogurt spiced with curry powder, tarragon, prepared mustard, and chives. Or try some Pritikin brand vinaigrette or creamy Italian dressing.

You can always add some millet or other grain to bolster the fiber content, too—and make your sandwich filling go farther. In Chapter 13 you'll find recipes for Salmon Pâté, as well as Pita-Bread Pizza and Lebanese Tabbouli Salad. Our recipes aren't only good in themselves—once you catch on to the principles behind them, you'll start coming up with your own. While you're chopping the white of an egg for a tuna salad, you'll realize you can have an egg-white salad, too. Speaking of egg whites, how about an egg-white omelet? They're delicious with any vegetable filling, like mushrooms, peppers, and onions, with Pritikin brand Mexican sauce, or even with a dollop of no-sugar-added jam, as a quick hot snack or dessert.

You can even make a hearty, satisfying potato salad: Cube or slice cold cooked potatoes and mix with our Mock Sour Cream recipe (see p. 268) or nonfat yogurt as well as chopped vegetables, herbs, and spices. For other snack ideas—including "portable" munchies like Tortilla Chips—see the recipes in Chapter 13.

SWEETS

These are often the things the would-be "dieter" frets most about having to give up. But since, as you know, you're not going on a "diet," we're not going to tell you to stay *away* from anything. There's so much in the repertoire of the Pritikin plan that will satisfy your sweet tooth—and, as you wake up to the subtleties of foods that haven't been blasted by an overdose of refined sugar, you'll find a natural sweetness not only in fruits such as oranges and peaches (where you'd expect to find it), but even in a slice of fresh whole-wheat bread, a bowl of undoctored hot cereal, and baked yams.

But that's not what we really mean by sweets—you'll have plenty of undeniably sweet food, don't worry! Pritikin brand fruit spreads are great on toast or muffins, and can also be melted for a terrific pancake syrup. Pureed fresh fruit or mashed and whipped bananas are also great on toast instead of jam or jelly. Unsweetened carob powder mixed with apple juice concentrate can even substitute for chocolate or cocoa in some recipes. And as we suggested earlier, you can make your own "sodas" by juicing fresh fruits and adding sparkling mineral water—or just by squeezing some citrus juice into salt-free seltzer or mineral water.

The heady aroma of spices such as cinnamon, nutmeg, vanilla, allspice, mace, ginger, and cardamom will make your food smell, and taste, sweet. And, of course, consult the many creative dessert recipes in Chapter 13, ranging from Yogurt Parfait to Cheesecake (which has a blueberry variation). It's amazing how many wonderful alternatives you can find to America's passion, ice cream: Frozen bananas that have been run through a blender or juicer taste exactly like the best soft-serve ice cream you've ever had (see our recipe for Banana "Ice Cream" on page 258); look, too, for frozen *nonfat* yogurt, which is becoming more widely available.

LABEL LOGIC: WATCHING FOR FAT, SALT, AND SUGAR

The foods you don't prepare from scratch, the ones you pick up for the sake of convenience or out of curiosity, or just because you like them—all the cereals, grains, breads, and pastas, the jams, and the prepared sauces and vegetables in the market—they all have invaluable nutrition information right on their labels. But because label reading takes some skill (there could be some hidden surprises in store), let's go over a few basic rules. The best information will be in

HOW TO CALCULATE THE PERCENTAGE OF CALORIES FROM FAT

While labels list fat content according to weight, a more useful reference is the percentage of total calories from fat in a given food. The Pritikin Lifetime Eating Plan derives approximately 10 percent of its calories from fat, 10 to 15 percent of its calories from protein, and 75 to 80 percent of its calories from carbohydrates. To stay within these guidelines, choose foods in which the fat content is no greater than 15 percent of total calories—you can still maintain an average intake of 10 percent since many foods are well under 10 percent total calories from fat. The exception to this 15 percent general rule is the high-protein category, where the amounts are controlled and the upper limit is 34 percent of calories from fat (and 90 milligrams of cholesterol) for all items. The only exception to the 34 percent upper limit is high-fat fish, such as salmon, which contains more than 34 percent fat.

Here's how to use the information on a standard food label to calculate the percentage of a food's total calories from fat. We'll use whole milk as an example.

Whole Milk

Serving Size:	1 cup
Calories:	160
Protein:	8 grams
Fat:	9 grams
Carbohydrates:	11 grams

the nutritional section of the label, where it tells the amounts of fat, cholesterol, and sodium contained in the product, so you can maintain the guidelines of the Pritikin Lifetime Eating Plan. It can come as quite a shock to learn just how much unhealthy food is passed off as "natural" or "wholesome" (even in health-food stores), so do take careful note of the following. You may not be able to judge a food by its "cover"—a slick label can fool you at first glance. But you *can* judge it by reading its list of ingredients, and it won't take long for you to become a pro at picking out what's good for you and what isn't.

The first thing to know about labels is that ingredients are always

Each gram of fat contains 9 calories (each gram of carbohydrate or protein contains 4 calories). To do the calculation, simply multiply the grams of fat by 9, and divide by the total calories. Then multiply by 100 to express your answer in percentage form.

For example:

(1) 9 grams of fat × 9 = 81 calories from fat
(2) 81 ÷ 160 = .51
(3) .51 × 100 = 51%

Thus, 51 percent of the calories in whole milk come from fat, although only about 4 percent of the weight of whole milk is fat. Here are three other listings of approximate fat content both by weight and by percentage of total calories:

	Percentage Fat by Weight	Percentage Fat by Calories
2% low-fat milk	2%	33%
1% low-fat milk	1%	19%
Nonfat (skim) milk	Less than 1%	Not more than 5%

listed in decreasing order of weight: The first item listed is the largest amount by weight.

Fats. High-fat ingredients go by the following names: butter, egg yolk, shortening, margarine, mayonnaise, lard, tallow, suet, "schmaltz" (chicken or goose fat), hydrogenated or partially hydrogenated vegetable shortening, vegetable oils (olive, canola, peanut, corn, safflower, soybean, coconut, and palm), monoglycerides, diglycerides, or triglycerides (the chemical name for oils and fats).

Hydrogenated fats (margarine is an example) start out as vegetable oils and are made solid by the addition of hydrogen. (Saturated fats, which are solid at room temperature, are saturated with hydrogen already in their natural state.) Animal fats, such as bacon fat, butter, and lard, are solid at room temperature and are composed mainly of saturated fatty acids. Vegetable oils, such as peanut, corn, and sunflower oils, are liquids at room temperature and consist primarily of polyunsaturated and/or monounsaturated fatty acids. Palm oil, coconut oil, and cocoa butter (the fat in chocolate) are vegetable fats that in their natural state are already highly saturated, thus making them, like animal fats, the worst offenders. While vegetable fats and oils contain no cholesterol (animal fats, of course, do), some have a powerful ability to raise blood cholesterol levels and promote other serious illnesses as well when consumed in the amounts typical of most Western diets.

Sodium. Sodium will also crop up in a bewildering variety of forms; the most common, of course, is sodium chloride (NaCl), table salt. Other ingredients that contain sodium include sea salt, kelp, baking powder, baking soda, monosodium glutamate (MSG), sodium saccharin, sodium nitrate, and sodium propionate.

Seasonings and condiments that are best avoided because of their high sodium content include onion, garlic, and celery salt; most commercial ketchups, chili sauces, and barbecue sauces; and cooking wines (regular wine may be used for cooking). Do keep on the lookout for low-sodium versions of chili sauce, barbecue sauce, and "imitation" ketchup—they're all available. (Real ketchup must be 20 percent sugar by weight, according to its "product identity.") If you use prepared mustards or even tamari or sodium-reduced soy sauce, use small amounts, because they, too, are relatively salty. And as you would with canned beans that contain salt, be sure to rinse such canned foods as capers, artichoke hearts, and chili peppers in lots of water to get rid of as much excess salt as possible. Once you've adjusted to a lower-salt diet, all of these foods will taste better after a "bath"!

Sugar. We've already mentioned the suffix "-ose": It signals sugar, as in sucrose, lactose, glucose, fructose, and the like.

Ingredients to be aware of include high-fructose corn syrup (and all of the other "-oses"), corn or grape sugar, corn or grape sweetener, maple sugar, cane sugar, brown sugar, barley malt, malted barley, rice syrup, raw sugar, sorghum, molasses, honey, sorbitol, and mannitol. Remember, for healthy individuals a little added sugar does not present the same health risks as added fats. Artificial sweeteners are best avoided—saccharin because animal studies have shown a link to cancer, and aspartame because its long-term effects simply aren't known yet. Artificial sweeteners may also increase your appetite for sweets.

The information we've laid out in this chapter isn't meant to bewilder you, and you certainly don't have to memorize it all before you go to the store (you might want to take some notes with you the first couple of times, however). What we want is for you to see, first of all, the many specific ways you can make eating on the Pritikin Lifetime Eating Plan a real pleasure *and* a convenience, and then for you to become aware of certain foods and ingredients that may be advertised as healthy but just aren't. Armed with these facts, and (we hope) inspired by the good food you can now start to make in your own kitchen, you can set up the right nutritional base at home—a place to treat yourself as beneficially as you can, and to learn as you go along. As you grow in self-confidence on the Lifetime Eating Plan, your whole perspective on food and health will inevitably change—and this will affect what you do outside your kitchen, too.

But before we send you out of the kitchen—and don't worry, we will (see Chapters 14 and 15 on going out to eat, and eating during holidays and when you travel)—let's move on to the menus and recipes we've been promising, so you can see—and taste—for yourself: the Pritikin plan means terrific food!

CHAPTER 13

Menus and Recipes

Sherried Pea Soup . . . Teriyaki Chicken . . . pasta with our Marinara Sauce . . . Cheesecake with a blueberry variation. *Blueberry cheesecake?* Yes! The Pritikin program's 21-day menu plan sets you up for three weeks of not only the healthiest eating you could want but the most delicious as well. From breakfast to dinner, it's an abundance of appetizers, entrees, snacks, and desserts you probably never expected to find: everything from Artichoke Pâté to Yogurt Parfait—and more! Here's where you find out exactly how to prepare them, *and* how simple most of our recipes are (we know you won't start a new food program if it means tackling complicated cooking procedures). Many of the dishes on the 21-day plan can be made in a flash, and you'll discover that even the more elaborate dishes end up *looking* harder to make than they really are.

The cooking methods we use are, in fact, ones with which you're no doubt familiar already. Here's a rundown:

Baking, or oven cooking. Cooking in an oven at a low temperature (200–300 degrees Fahrenheit), a moderate temperature (325–400 degrees), or a hot temperature (400–500 degrees).

Boiling. Cooking in water at 212 degrees or over.

Microwaving. Cooking in a microwave oven. The appearance, flavor, and nutrient values of foods are enhanced in microwave cooking, while cooking time is greatly reduced.

Steaming. Cooking over boiling water or in such a manner that steam passes around the food. Steaming is one of the better preparation methods: Because the food does not come in direct contact with the water, it retains more of its nutrients.

184

Pressure-cooking. Using a pressure cooker, food is cooked under pressure at high temperatures, for a shorter period of time than with most other methods.

Braising. "Browning" food in a small amount of stock, then cooking, covered, in the juices or in a small amount of added liquid.

Pan-broiling. Cooking in a heated iron skillet or griddle, without oils or fats.

Simmering. Cooking slowly in hot liquid, over very low heat, either to make tender or to develop flavor.

Broiling. Cooking by direct exposure to heat, either under or over a gas flame or electric heating element, or between two heated surfaces, or over hot coals (as on a barbecue, open grill, or rotisserie).

EQUIPPING YOUR HEALTHY KITCHEN

You'll also find that you won't have to go out and buy armloads of special paraphernalia to cook healthy foods. Most of what you'll need you probably already own. As you'll see from the following list, appliances, cookware, and utensils are fairly standard—with an emphasis on nonstick items. This list is simply for your reference. You do not have to purchase anything, but these items might make your food preparation quicker. You probably have most of these things in your kitchen already, but if you're thinking about making some purchases, bear these tips in mind:

- When buying nonstick skillets, do invest in the *best* you can find: They'll last you for many years, so it's worth it. Nonstick cookware is recommended because you won't have to use fats to keep your food from sticking.
- Good knives with high-quality blades are a must, too, and not just because they're easier to use: They're also safer. A well-sharpened knife will cut vegetables, meats, or breads easily; a dull one is far more apt to slip off the food and cut you instead.
- A food processor is a great tool for making food preparation easier. Delicious recipes such as Banana "Ice Cream," Salmon Pâté, and Mock Sour Cream can all be made quickly. Extra blades may also help with cutting vegetables in different sizes and shapes.

COOKWARE AND BAKEWARE

Assorted sizes of nonstick skillets
Assorted nonstick bakeware such as muffin pans, square pans, cookie sheets, tube pans
Assorted glassware such as pie plates and casseroles
Assorted pots, including a stock pot

APPLIANCES

Food processor with extra blades
Blender
Electric mixer
Nonstick wok
Air popcorn popper
Microwave oven

UTENSILS

Depending on your preference, you may wish to expand on these choices or focus on just a few essentials.
A good set of sharp knives: assorted sizes
Peeler
Citrus peel zester (optional)
Mixing bowls: assorted sizes
Rubber spatulas
Plastic spatulas
Long-handled slotted spoon (plastic or metal)
Long-handled fork
Assorted wooden spoons
Colander
Strainer, about 5 or 6 inches in diameter
Kitchen scale (optional)
Timer
Garlic press
Gravy strainer
Dry measuring cups
Liquid measuring cups
Measuring spoons
Grater
Cutting board
Ice cube trays
Juicer

Steamer basket
Wire whisk

MISCELLANEOUS

Parchment paper
Food-release spray
Cheesecloth
Plastic storage/freezer containers for grains, pastas, and leftovers

BE CREATIVE!

What we hope is that the following menu plans and recipes will spark your *own* food ideas—once you've mastered the principles, there's no reason you can't create your own recipes and food combinations. We think you'll find the recipes on the following pages versatile and exciting, and you can certainly mix and match these dishes to make a plan for far longer than three weeks. Be creative!

The menu plans are designed for the 1,000- and 1,200-calorie plans. If you are not looking to lose weight quickly, you will not need to watch portion sizes except for high-protein and dairy exchanges. Try some of these delicious recipes, but add potatoes, bread, other complex carbohydrates, fruits, and vegetables to your menu plans. And remember that any recipe with an asterisk (*) is included in this book.

These recipes come with a detailed breakdown that includes the number of complex-carbohydrate, vegetable, fruit, high-protein, and/or dairy exchanges in a given portion of each dish, along with the sodium content, total calories, amount of cholesterol, and percentage of calories from fat. You won't need to check all this information every time you cook—as we said in Chapter 11, simply by eating the recommended numbers of servings you'll get optimal nutrition *and* meet the goals of the Pritikin plan. But these nutritional values will help you when you branch out on your own to create new dishes. You'll have an idea of which foods to emphasize, and in what combination, for maximum nutritional benefit.

Tested and perfected at the Pritikin Longevity Center kitchens, these recipes offer an imaginative, uncomplicated approach to the food you'll want to make your own. You can use these recipes with the menu plans for faster weight loss, or just try any of them anytime. You don't have to be concerned with weight loss to sample these appetizing meals! Whether you're cooking for one or for a crowd, you'll find a bounty of wonderful foods to satisfy everyone. And if you do cook for others, you can be sure of one thing: They may never know how healthful your food is, but they'll have no doubt about how delicious it is!

Menus

KEY TO EXCHANGES

CC = Complex carbohydrates
FR = Fruit
V = Vegetable
D = Dairy
HP = High protein

Recipes are provided for those items marked with an asterisk (*).
For more information on the Exchange System, see Chapter 11.

DAY 1

Exchanges	Portion	1,000 Calories	For 1,200 Calories Add:
		BREAKFAST	
$\frac{1}{4}$ D, $\frac{1}{4}$ V	1 serving	Mexican Eggs*	
1 CC	1 tortilla	Steamed corn tortilla	
1 FR	1 cup	Fresh papaya	
1 D	8 oz.	Nonfat milk	
		Chamomile tea	
		MORNING SNACK	
$\frac{1}{2}$ CC	1	Pritikin brand rice cake, with 1 tsp. sugarless apple butter	2 Pritikin brand rice cakes; 1 nectarine
		LUNCH	
1 CC, $\frac{1}{4}$ D	1 cup	Sherried Pea Soup*	1 additional sliced tomato
1 V	1 medium	Sliced tomato	
$\frac{1}{2}$ CC	2	Rye crackers	
2 V	2 cups	Salad greens	
	2 Tbsp.	Pritikin brand dressing	
1 FR	$\frac{3}{4}$ cup	Fresh or frozen boysenberries	
$\frac{1}{2}$ D	3 oz.	Nonfat yogurt (mix with fruit)	
		AFTERNOON SNACK	
$1\frac{3}{4}$ V	$1\frac{3}{4}$ cups	Raw vegetables	Additional cup raw vegetables
		DINNER	
1 V	1 small	Steamed artichoke	
1 FR	1 cup	Fresh Apple Soda*	
$3\frac{1}{2}$ oz. HP	$3\frac{1}{2}$ oz.	Teriyaki Steak*	
1 V	1 cup	Green-Bean Salad*	
1 CC	1 medium	Baked potato	
Totals		1,000	1,200
CC		4	5
FR		3	4
V		7	9
D		2	2
HP		$3\frac{1}{2}$ oz.	$3\frac{1}{2}$ oz.

DAY 2

Exchanges	Portion	1,000 Calories	For 1,200 Calories Add:
		BREAKFAST	
1 CC, 1 FR	$\frac{1}{2}$ cup	Peach Oatmeal*	
1 D	8 oz.	Nonfat milk	
	6 oz.	Hot grain beverage	
		MORNING SNACK	
1 CC	$\frac{1}{2}$ bagel	Whole-wheat bagel	$\frac{1}{3}$ cantaloupe
		LUNCH	
1 CC, $1\frac{1}{2}$ V	1 medium	Baked potato with	Whole-wheat, French, or
	$\frac{1}{2}$ cup	Marinara Sauce*	sourdough
$1\frac{1}{2}$ V	$1\frac{1}{2}$ cups	Salad greens	roll
1 FR	$\frac{3}{4}$ cup	Fresh fruit cup	
		AFTERNOON SNACK	
1 V	1 cup	Raw broccoli and cauliflower with Pritikin brand ranch dressing	
		DINNER	
3 oz. HP, $\frac{1}{2}$ D	1 serving	Chicken Curry*	
1 V	$\frac{1}{2}$ cup	Steamed asparagus	Additional $\frac{1}{2}$ cup
2 V	2 cups	Tossed green salad with red wine vinegar	asparagus; additional
1 CC	$\frac{1}{2}$ cup	Wild rice	cup green
$\frac{1}{2}$ D	4 oz.	Nonfat milk	salad
1 FR	1 Tbsp.	Chutney* or	
	1 oz.	Grapes	
Totals		1,000	1,200
CC		4	5
FR		3	4
V		7	9
D		2	2
HP		3 oz.	3 oz.

DAY 3

Exchanges	Portion	1,000 Calories	For 1,200 Calories Add:
		BREAKFAST	
2 CC, $\frac{1}{2}$ FR	2 slices	Banana French Toast*	Additional slice Banana French Toast
$\frac{1}{2}$ FR	$\frac{1}{4}$ cup	Fruit Syrup*	
1 D	8 oz.	Nonfat milk	
		MORNING SNACK	
1 V	1 cup	Red and green pepper strips	
		LUNCH	
1 CC	$\frac{1}{2}$ cup	Whole-wheat pasta	1 cup raw
3 V	1 serving	Ratatouille*	vegetable
$\frac{1}{2}$ FR	$1\frac{1}{4}$ cup	Fresh strawberries	salad
1 D	6 oz.	with nonfat yogurt	
		AFTERNOON SNACK	
1 V	6 oz.	Unsalted vegetable juice	2 medium apricots
		DINNER	
$3\frac{1}{2}$ HP, 1 FR, 1 CC	1 serving	Cranberry-Glazed Chicken Breast with Whole-Grain Stuffing*	
1 V	$\frac{1}{2}$ cup	Brussels sprouts	
1 V	$\frac{1}{2}$ cup	Carrot Salad*	Additional $\frac{1}{2}$ cup Carrot Salad

Totals		1,000	1,200
CC		4	5
FR		3	4
V		7	9
D		2	2
HP		$3\frac{1}{2}$ oz.	$3\frac{1}{2}$ oz.

DAY 4

Exchanges	Portion	1,000 Calories	For 1,200 Calories Add:
		BREAKFAST	
1 CC	$\frac{1}{2}$ cup	Spoon-size wheat-biscuit cereal	$\frac{1}{2}$ whole-wheat
1 FR	$\frac{1}{2}$	Ripe sliced banana	bagel with 2 tsp. Pritikin
1 D	8 oz.	Nonfat milk	brand
	8 oz.	Linden-flower tea	blueberry fruit spread
		MORNING SNACK	
1 CC	2	Pritikin brand 7-grain rice cakes	
		LUNCH	
1 CC	$\frac{1}{2}$ can	Pritikin brand lentil soup	1 cup carrot
3 V	3 cups	Tossed salad with herb vinegar dressing	sticks; 6 oz. unsalted vege-
1 FR	1 large	Sliced kiwi	table juice
		AFTERNOON SNACK	
1 D	6 oz.	Nonfat plain yogurt, sweetened with 1 tsp. Pritikin brand blueberry fruit spread	12 large cherries
		DINNER—RESTAURANT	
$3\frac{1}{2}$ oz. HP	$3\frac{1}{2}$ oz.	Broiled halibut or poached salmon	
1 V	1	Steamed artichoke	
1 CC	1 small	Baked potato	
1 V	$\frac{1}{2}$ cup	Mushrooms "sautéed" in wine	
2 V	2 cups	Salad—Belgian endive, asparagus, yellow pepper	
1 FR	$\frac{3}{4}$ cup	Raspberries	
Totals		1,000	1,200
CC		4	5
FR		3	4
V		7	9
D		2	2
HP		$3\frac{1}{2}$ oz.	$3\frac{1}{2}$ oz.

DAY 5

Exchanges	Portion	1,000 Calories	For 1,200 Calories Add:
		BREAKFAST	
1 CC, $\frac{1}{2}$ D, $\frac{1}{2}$ FR	1 serving	Hot Nugget Cereal*	1 slice whole-wheat toast
$\frac{1}{2}$ FR	1 Tbsp.	Raisins	
$\frac{1}{2}$ D	4 oz.	Nonfat milk	
		MORNING SNACK	
1 FR	$1\frac{1}{4}$ cups	Watermelon	
		LUNCH—ITALIAN RESTAURANT	
2 CC, 1 V	$1\frac{1}{2}$ cups	Spaghetti with fresh tomato and basil	
2 V	2 cups	Fresh green salad with lemon juice	1 cup fresh fruit in season
		AFTERNOON SNACK	
1 V	1 cup	Raw broccoli and cauliflower	1 cup sliced tomatoes and cucumbers
		DINNER	
3 oz. HP, 1 FR, 1 V	1 serving	Pineapple Chicken*	
1 CC	$\frac{1}{3}$ cup	Brown rice	
1 V	$\frac{1}{2}$ cup	Steamed pea pods	Additional $\frac{1}{2}$ cup pea pods
1 V	1 cup	Salad greens	
1 D	6 oz.	Nonfat yogurt with 1 tsp. vanilla, cinnamon	

Totals	1,000	1,200
CC	4	5
FR	3	4
V	7	9
D	2	2
HP	3 oz.	3 oz.

DAY 6

Exchanges	Portion	1,000 Calories	For 1,200 Calories Add:
		BREAKFAST	
1 CC, $\frac{1}{2}$ FR	1	Oat-Bran Muffin*	
$\frac{2}{3}$ D	4 oz.	Nonfat yogurt	
		Chamomile tea	
		MORNING SNACK	
1 FR	1 medium	Fresh peach, sliced	1 cup assorted raw vegetables
		LUNCH	
1 CC, $\frac{1}{2}$ D, 2 V	1 pizza	Pita-Bread Pizza*	
2 V	$\frac{2}{3}$ cup	Mushroom Antipasto*	Additional $\frac{1}{2}$ cup Mushroom Antipasto
$\frac{1}{2}$ CC	1	Breadstick	
		AFTERNOON SNACK	
1 V	1 cup	Cherry tomatoes, stuffed	$1\frac{1}{4}$ cups
$\frac{1}{2}$ D	2 Tbsp.	with Yogurt Cheese*	watermelon
		DINNER	
$3\frac{1}{2}$ oz. HP	$3\frac{1}{2}$ oz.	Poached salmon, with	1
$\frac{1}{3}$ D	$\frac{1}{4}$ cup	Dill Sauce*	whole-wheat roll
2 V	1 cup	Steamed Italian squash and carrots	
1 CC	$\frac{1}{3}$ cup	Brown rice	
$1\frac{1}{2}$ FR, $\frac{1}{2}$ CC	1 slice	Jewel-of-Fruit Pie*	
Totals		1,000	1,200
CC		4	5
FR		3	4
V		7	9
D		2	2
HP		$3\frac{1}{2}$ oz.	$3\frac{1}{2}$ oz.

DAY 7

Exchanges	Portion	1,000 Calories	For 1,200 Calories Add:
		BREAKFAST	
1 CC	$\frac{1}{2}$ cup	Wheat flakes	1 slice whole-wheat toast with 1 tsp. Pritikin brand fruit spread
$1\frac{1}{4}$ D	10 oz.	Nonfat milk	
1 FR	$\frac{1}{2}$ medium	Banana	
		MORNING SNACK	
2 V	2 cups	Carrot and jicama strips	2 plums
		LUNCH	
2 CC, 1 V	1	Vegetarian submarine: wheat bun with 1 cup raw vegetables and Pritikin brand Italian dressing or mustard	
1 V	6 oz.	Unsalted vegetable juice	
1 FR	$\frac{1}{2}$ cup	Kiwi and orange slices	
		AFTERNOON SNACK	
2 V	1 cup	Chinese Tomato Soup*	
1 CC	2	Pritikin brand sesame rice cakes	
		DINNER	
1 CC, $\frac{3}{4}$ D, 2 V	1 serving	Cannelloni*	Additional cup tossed salad; 1 whole-wheat roll; additional $\frac{1}{2}$ cup zucchini
1 V	$\frac{1}{2}$ cup	Steamed zucchini	
1 FR	$\frac{1}{8}$	Honeydew melon	
1 V	1 cup	Tossed salad	

Totals	1,000	1,200
CC	5	7
FR	3	4
V	10	12
D	2	2
HP	0	0

DAY 8

Exchanges	Portion	1,000 Calories	For 1,200 Calories Add:
		BREAKFAST	
1 CC	2	Latkes (Potato Pancakes)*	
1 FR	$\frac{1}{2}$ cup	Hot Cinnamon Applesauce*	
1 D	8 oz.	Nonfat milk	
		MORNING SNACK	
$\frac{1}{2}$ CC	1	Pritikin brand 7-grain rice cake	1 tangerine
1 V	1 cup	Assorted raw vegetables	
		LUNCH—MEXICAN RESTAURANT	
1 CC, 1 oz. HP, $\frac{1}{2}$ V	1	Soft chicken taco: steamed corn tortilla, chicken, vegetables, salsa	$\frac{1}{2}$ cup *frijoles de olla* (boiled beans)
2 V	2 cups	Tossed salad with salsa or lemon	
1 FR		Pineapple juice spritzer: $\frac{1}{2}$ cup pineapple juice, $\frac{1}{2}$ cup seltzer, ice	
		AFTERNOON SNACK	
$\frac{1}{2}$ D, $\frac{1}{2}$ V	1 cup	Cold Cucumber Soup*	1 Steamed artichoke
		DINNER	
2 oz. HP, $\frac{1}{2}$ CC	1 serving	Mini Meatballs*	
$1\frac{1}{2}$ V	$\frac{1}{2}$ cup	Marinara Sauce*	
1 CC	$\frac{1}{2}$ cup	Whole-wheat pasta	
$1\frac{1}{2}$ V	$1\frac{1}{2}$ cups	Vegetable salad with Pritikin brand creamy Italian dressing	Additional cup salad
$\frac{1}{2}$ D, 1 FR	1 serving	Flan*	
Totals		1,000	1,200
CC		4	5
FR		3	4
V		7	9
D		2	2
HP		3 oz.	3 oz.

DAY 9

Exchanges	Portion	1,000 Calories	For 1,200 Calories Add:
		BREAKFAST	
2 CC	$\frac{1}{2}$ cup	Granola*	
1 FR	$\frac{3}{4}$ cup	Blueberries	
1 D	8 oz.	Nonfat milk	
		MORNING SNACK	
1 V	1 cup	Assorted raw vegetables	Additional cup vegetables; 1 medium apple
		LUNCH	
1 CC, 1 V	1 cup	Lebanese Tabbouli Salad*	1 whole-wheat pita
1 V	1 cup	Green and red pepper strips	
1 D	6 oz.	Nonfat yogurt	
1 FR	$\frac{1}{8}$	Honeydew melon	
		AFTERNOON SNACK	
1 V	1	Steamed artichoke	Additional artichoke
		DINNER—RESTAURANT	
$3\frac{1}{2}$ oz. HP	$3\frac{1}{2}$ oz.	Filet of sole, broiled with lemon and herbs	
1 V	$\frac{1}{2}$ cup	Steamed baby carrots	
2 V	2 cups	Tossed green salad	
1 CC	1 medium	Baked potato	
1 FR	$\frac{1}{2}$ cup	Fresh fruit in season	
Totals		1,000	1,200
CC		4	5
FR		3	4
V		7	9
D		2	2
HP		$3\frac{1}{2}$ oz.	$3\frac{1}{2}$ oz.

DAY 10

Exchanges	Portion	1,000 Calories	For 1,200 Calories Add:
		BREAKFAST	
2 CC	1	Pritikin brand English muffin	
1 FR	$\frac{1}{3}$	Cantaloupe	
1 D	8 oz.	Cafe Olé*	
		MORNING SNACK	
1 FR	1 medium	Orange	
		LUNCH	
1 CC, $\frac{1}{2}$ D, 1 V	1	English tea sandwich: $\frac{1}{2}$ pita with Artichoke Pâté* and sliced cucumber	
1 V	1 cup	Fresh vegetable salad	Additional cup salad; 1 medium apple
		AFTERNOON SNACK	
1 V	1 cup	Cherry tomatoes	1 whole-wheat roll
		DINNER	
$3\frac{1}{2}$ oz. HP, 1 FR, 1 V	1 serving	Teriyaki Chicken*	
1 CC, 1 V	$\frac{3}{4}$ cup	Oriental Rice*	
2 V	1 cup	Bok choy (or baby bok choy), steamed	Additional $\frac{1}{2}$ cup bok choy, steamed
$\frac{1}{2}$ D	4 oz.	Nonfat milk	
Totals		1,000	1,200
CC		4	5
FR		3	4
V		7	9
D		2	2
HP		$3\frac{1}{2}$ oz.	$3\frac{1}{2}$ oz.

DAY 11

Exchanges	Portion	1,000 Calories	For 1,200 Calories Add:
		BREAKFAST	
1 CC, 1 D, $\frac{1}{2}$ FR	1	Cheese Blintz*	$\frac{1}{2}$ grapefruit
$\frac{1}{2}$ FR	$\frac{1}{4}$ cup	Fruit Syrup*	
		MORNING SNACK	
1 V	6 oz.	Unsalted vegetable juice	
		LUNCH	
2 V	1 cup	Gazpacho*	1 medium
1 CC	10 chips	Tortilla Chips*	baked potato
1 V	1 cup	Steamed broccoli with lemon	with salsa
1 FR	$1\frac{1}{4}$ cups	Watermelon	
		AFTERNOON SNACK	
1 V	1 cup	Carrot and celery sticks	Additional
1 CC	$\frac{1}{2}$	Whole-wheat pita	cup vegetables
		DINNER	
3 oz. HP	1 serving	Fish in Lime Sauce*	1 cup
2 V	1 cup	Steamed asparagus	vegetable
1 CC	$\frac{1}{2}$ cup	Cracked bulgur wheat	salad
1 FR	$\frac{1}{2}$ cup	Rainbow fruit cup (kiwi, banana, fresh berries)	
1 D	8 oz.	Nonfat milk	
Totals		1,000	1,200
CC		4	5
FR		3	4
V		7	9
D		2	2
HP		3 oz.	3 oz.

DAY 12

Exchanges	Portion	1,000 Calories	For 1,200 Calories Add:
		BREAKFAST	
1 CC, $\frac{1}{2}$ V	1 serving	Huevos Rancheros*	
1 D	8 oz.	Nonfat milk	
1 FR	$\frac{3}{4}$ cup	Fresh pineapple	
		MORNING SNACK	
1 FR	15	Grapes	
		LUNCH	
2 CC	1 cup	Pritikin brand whole-wheat spaghetti	Additional $\frac{1}{2}$ cup
1 V	$\frac{1}{3}$ cup	Marinara Sauce*	spaghetti;
1 V	$\frac{1}{2}$ cup	Eggplant, steamed	additional $\frac{1}{3}$
1 FR	$\frac{3}{4}$ cup	Fresh boysenberries	cup Marinara
1 D	6 oz.	Nonfat yogurt (mix with boysenberries)	Sauce
		AFTERNOON SNACK	
1 V	1 cup	Fresh green salad with Pritikin brand dressing	1 medium peach
		DINNER—CHINESE RESTAURANT	
3 oz. HP, $3\frac{1}{2}$ V	$2\frac{1}{2}$ cups	Moo goo gai pan (chicken with Oriental vegetables)	Additional $\frac{1}{2}$ cup
1 CC	$\frac{1}{3}$ cup	Steamed rice	vegetables
	8 oz.	Herbal tea	
Totals		1,000	1,200
CC		4	5
FR		3	4
V		7	9
D		2	2
HP		3 oz.	3 oz.

DAY 13

Exchanges	Portion	1,000 Calories	For 1,200 Calories Add:
		BREAKFAST	
2 CC	1 bagel	Whole-wheat bagel	Additional $\frac{1}{2}$ whole-wheat bagel with 1 tsp. Pritikin brand fruit spread
1 FR	$\frac{1}{2}$ medium	Banana	
		MORNING SNACK	
1 FR	$\frac{1}{8}$	Honeydew melon	
		LUNCH	
1 CC	1	Whole-wheat roll	$\frac{3}{4}$ cup fresh pineapple
3 V	3 cups	Spinach/mushroom salad: fresh spinach, mushrooms, green/red pepper, lemon juice	
1 V	1	Steamed artichoke with lemon	Additional artichoke
		AFTERNOON SNACK	
1 D	6 oz.	Nonfat yogurt, sweetened with 1 tsp. Pritikin brand fruit spread	
		DINNER	
$3\frac{1}{2}$ oz. HP	$3\frac{1}{2}$ oz.	Roast breast of turkey	
1 V	1 medium	Broiled tomato slices with basil	
2 V	2 cups	Assorted raw vegetable salad with Pritikin brand dressing	Additional cup salad
1 CC	$\frac{1}{2}$ cup	Green peas and pearl onions	
1 FR, 1 D	1 serving	Yogurt Parfait*	
Totals		1,000	1,200
CC		4	5
FR		3	4
V		7	9
D		2	2
HP		$3\frac{1}{2}$ oz.	$3\frac{1}{2}$ oz.

DAY 14

Exchanges	Portion	1,000 Calories	For 1,200 Calories Add:
		BREAKFAST	
1 CC	$\frac{1}{2}$ cup	Maple Oatmeal*	Additional $\frac{1}{2}$
1 FR	2 Tbsp.	Raisins	cup Maple
1 D	8 oz.	Nonfat milk	Oatmeal
		MORNING SNACK	
1 FR	1	Nectarine	
$\frac{1}{2}$ D	3 oz.	Nonfat yogurt	
		LUNCH—RESTAURANT	
1 CC	1 medium	Baked potato with	
1 V	$\frac{1}{2}$ cup	Salsa or marinara sauce	
2 V	2 cups	Salad bar	
1 FR	1 medium	Fresh fruit in season	
		Mineral water with lime	
		AFTERNOON SNACK	
1 V	1 cup	Green and red pepper strips	Additional
1 CC	$\frac{1}{2}$	Whole-wheat pita	cup pepper strips
		DINNER	
$3\frac{1}{2}$ oz. HP	1 serving	Chicken à l'Orange*	
2 V	1 cup	Steamed broccoli	Additional
1 CC, $\frac{1}{2}$ D	$\frac{2}{3}$ cup	Scalloped Potatoes*	cup salad;
1 V	1 cup	Tossed green salad	baked apple
Totals		1,000	1,200
CC		4	5
FR		3	4
V		7	9
D		2	2
HP		$3\frac{1}{2}$ oz.	$3\frac{1}{2}$ oz.

DAY 15

Exchanges	Portion	1,000 Calories	For 1,200 Calories Add:
		BREAKFAST	
1 CC, $\frac{1}{2}$ V	$\frac{1}{2}$	Egg on a Muffin*	Additional $\frac{1}{2}$
1 FR	$\frac{1}{2}$	Grapefruit	Egg on a
1 D	8 oz.	Nonfat milk	Muffin
		MORNING SNACK	
1 V	6 oz.	Unsalted vegetable juice	$\frac{1}{2}$ small mango
		LUNCH—BROWN-BAG LUNCH	
$1\frac{1}{2}$ oz. HP	$\frac{1}{4}$ cup	Salmon Pâté*	1 cup salad
1 CC	$\frac{1}{2}$	Whole-wheat pita	
1 V	1 cup	Assorted raw vegetables (tomatoes, onions, sprouts)	
1 FR	$1\frac{1}{4}$ cups	Fresh strawberries	
1 D	6 oz.	Nonfat yogurt	
		AFTERNOON SNACK	
1 CC	1 medium	Baked potato	
1 V	$\frac{1}{2}$ cup	Salsa	
		DINNER	
$1\frac{1}{2}$ oz. HP, 3 V	1 serving	Spicy Beef*	
1 CC	$\frac{1}{2}$ cup	Bulgur	
1 FR	$\frac{1}{2}$ cup	Kiwi and orange wedges	
	1 cup	Spiced Tea*	
$\frac{1}{2}$ V	$\frac{1}{2}$ cup	Vegetable salad	Additional $\frac{1}{2}$ cup salad
Totals		1,000	1,200
CC		4	5
FR		3	4
V		7	9
D		2	2
HP		3 oz.	3 oz.

DAY 16

Exchanges	Portion	1,000 Calories	For 1,200 Calories Add:
		BREAKFAST	
1 CC, 1 FR	2	Granola Date Bar*	
1 D	8 oz.	Nonfat milk	
		MORNING SNACK	
$\frac{1}{2}$ D, $\frac{1}{2}$ FR	1 serving	Piña Colada Frozen Yogurt*	
		LUNCH	
1 CC, 1 V	1 serving	Black-Bean Soup*	1 corn tortilla
$\frac{1}{4}$ D	$1\frac{1}{2}$ oz.	Top soup with nonfat yogurt	
2 V	2 cups	Fresh green salad	1 orange
1 V	$\frac{1}{2}$ cup	Salsa	
		AFTERNOON SNACK	
1 V	1 cup	Marinated Mushrooms*	Additional cup Marinated Mushrooms
		DINNER	
$3\frac{1}{2}$ oz. HP	$3\frac{1}{2}$ oz.	Scallops poached in white wine	1 tomato, sliced
2 V	1 cup	Yellow crookneck squash and brussels sprouts	
1 CC	$\frac{1}{3}$ cup	Sweet potato	
1 CC, $1\frac{1}{2}$ FR	1 piece	Apple-Date Cake*	
$\frac{1}{4}$ D	3 Tbsp.	Whoopee Topping*	
Totals		1,000	1,200
CC		4	5
FR		3	4
V		7	9
D		2	2
HP		$3\frac{1}{2}$ oz.	$3\frac{1}{2}$ oz.

DAY 17

Exchanges	Portion	1,000 Calories	For 1,200 Calories Add:
		BREAKFAST	
1 CC	1	Oatmeal Pancake*	1 additional
1 FR	$\frac{1}{2}$ cup	Hot Cinnamon Applesauce*	Oatmeal
1 D	8 oz.	Nonfat milk	Pancake
		MORNING SNACK	
1 FR	1 small	Pear	1 cup raw cauliflower
		LUNCH—CHINESE RESTAURANT	
1 CC	$\frac{1}{3}$ cup	Rice	
3 V	$1\frac{1}{2}$ cups	Steamed vegetables (called "Buddha's Delight" in many Chinese restaurants)	Additional $\frac{1}{2}$ cup vegetables; $\frac{3}{4}$ cup orange sections
		AFTERNOON SNACK	
2 V	2 cups	Raw vegetables with balsamic vinegar	
		DINNER	
$3\frac{1}{2}$ oz. HP	$3\frac{1}{2}$-oz.	Poached bass, with	
$\frac{1}{2}$ D	6 Tbsp.	Dill Sauce*	
2 V	2 cups	Cucumber Salad*	
1 CC	1 cup	Peas and onions	
1 CC	1 slice	Whole-wheat bread	
1 FR, $\frac{1}{2}$ D	1 serving	Strawberry-Yogurt Creme*	
Totals		1,000	1,200
CC		4	5
FR		3	4
V		7	9
D		2	2
HP		$3\frac{1}{2}$ oz.	$3\frac{1}{2}$ oz.

DAY 18

Exchanges	Portion	1,000 Calories	For 1,200 Calories Add:
		BREAKFAST	
1 CC	$\frac{1}{2}$ cup	Spoon-size wheat-biscuit cereal	
1 FR	$\frac{1}{2}$ medium	Banana	
1 D	8 oz.	Nonfat milk	
		MORNING SNACK	
1 CC	2	Pritikin brand rice cakes with 1 tsp. unsweetened apple butter	4 medium apricots
		LUNCH	
1 CC, 1 V	1 can ($7\frac{3}{8}$ oz.)	Pritikin brand minestrone soup	$\frac{1}{2}$ whole-wheat pita;
2 V	2 cups	Raw vegetable medley with Pritikin brand Italian dressing	additional cup
1 FR	$\frac{1}{2}$ cup	Unsweetened applesauce	vegetables
		AFTERNOON SNACK	
1 V	1 cup	Cherry tomatoes	1 cup tossed salad with herb vinegar
		DINNER	
$3\frac{1}{2}$ oz. HP, $\frac{1}{2}$ FR	1 serving	Chicken in Raspberry Marinade*	
3 V	$1\frac{1}{2}$ cups	Steamed baby carrots, mushrooms, and zucchini with lemon juice	
1 CC	$\frac{1}{3}$ cup	Brown and wild rice	
1 D, $\frac{1}{2}$ FR	2 servings	Cheesecake with blueberry variation*	
Totals		1,000	1,200
CC		4	5
FR		3	4
V		7	9
D		2	2
HP		$3\frac{1}{2}$ oz.	$3\frac{1}{2}$ oz.

DAY 19

Exchanges	Portion	1,000 Calories	For 1,200 Calories Add:
		BREAKFAST	
1 CC	$\frac{1}{2}$ cup	Cornflakes	Additional $\frac{1}{2}$
1 FR	$\frac{1}{2}$	Grapefruit	cup
1 D	8 oz.	Nonfat milk	cornflakes
		MORNING SNACK	
1 CC	$\frac{1}{2}$	Whole-wheat bagel	$\frac{1}{8}$ honeydew melon
		LUNCH	
1 CC, $\frac{1}{2}$ D, 2 V	1 pizza	Pita-Bread Pizza*	
1 V	1 cup	Lettuce and tomato salad	Additional
1 FR	1 medium	Apple	cup salad
$\frac{1}{2}$ D	3 oz.	Nonfat yogurt	
		AFTERNOON SNACK	
1 V	1 cup	Assorted raw vegetables	
		DINNER—RESTAURANT	
$3\frac{1}{2}$ oz. HP	$3\frac{1}{2}$ oz.	Seafood kabob	1 cup tossed
1 V	$\frac{1}{2}$ cup	Broccoli	salad;
2 V	2 cups	Salad with red wine vinegar	additional $\frac{1}{2}$
1 CC	2	Boiled new potatoes	cup broccoli
1 FR	$\frac{3}{4}$ cup	Fresh fruit cup	
Totals		1,000	1,200
CC		4	5
FR		3	4
V		7	10
D		2	2
HP		$3\frac{1}{2}$ oz.	$3\frac{1}{2}$ oz.

DAY 20

Exchanges	Portion	1,000 Calories	For 1,200 Calories Add:
		BREAKFAST	
1 D	1 serving	Cafe Olé*	
1 CC, 1 FR, $\frac{1}{2}$ D	1 serving	Banana Roll-up*	
		MORNING SNACK	
$1\frac{1}{2}$ FR	3 small	Plums	
		LUNCH—RESTAURANT	
$\frac{1}{2}$ oz. HP, 3 V	3 cups	Chef salad: $\frac{1}{2}$ oz. fresh turkey, assorted fresh vegetables, egg whites	
1 CC	4	Rye crackers, unsalted	1 medium peach
		AFTERNOON SNACK	
1 V	1 cup	Unsalted vegetable juice	1 cup jicama and celery
1 CC	6-inch ear	Corn on the cob	
		DINNER	
3 oz. HP, 1 V	1 serving	Red Snapper Veracruz*	1 cup green salad; 1
1 CC	$\frac{1}{3}$ cup	Wild rice	whole-wheat
2 V	1 cup	Carrot Salad*	roll
$\frac{1}{2}$ D, $\frac{1}{2}$ FR	$\frac{1}{2}$ cup	Frozen Blueberry Custard*	
__Totals__		__1,000__	__1,200__
CC		4	5
FR		3	4
V		7	9
D		2	2
HP		$3\frac{1}{2}$ oz.	$3\frac{1}{2}$ oz.

DAY 21

Exchanges	Portion	1,000 Calories	For 1,200 Calories Add:
		BREAKFAST	
1 CC	$\frac{1}{2}$ serving	Bagel Danish*	Additional $\frac{1}{3}$
1 FR	$\frac{1}{3}$	Cantaloupe	cantaloupe
1 D	8 oz.	Nonfat milk	
		MORNING SNACK	
2 V	2 cups	Broccoli and cauliflower florets	
		LUNCH	
$1\frac{1}{2}$ oz. HP, 1 V, $\frac{1}{2}$ FR	1 serving	Tuna Salad*	
1 CC	$\frac{1}{2}$	Whole-wheat pita	
1 V	1 cup	Tomatoes, sliced	
1 D	6 oz.	Nonfat yogurt	
$\frac{1}{2}$ FR	$\frac{3}{4}$ cup	Fresh strawberries (for yogurt)	
		AFTERNOON SNACK	
2 V	2 cups	Gazpacho*	
		DINNER	
2 V, 1 CC	1 serving	Vegetarian Moo Shoo*	Additional serving Vegetarian Moo Shoo with pancake
1 CC	$\frac{1}{3}$ cup	Brown rice	
1 FR	$\frac{1}{4}$ cup	Banana "Ice Cream"*	
Totals		1,000	1,200
CC		4	5
FR		3	4
V		8	10
D		2	2
HP		$1\frac{1}{2}$ oz.	$1\frac{1}{2}$ oz.

Recipes*
BREAKFAST AND BRUNCH

* The abbreviation "mg" at the ends of the recipes means "milligrams"; the sodium and cholesterol contents are per serving. "% fat" means the percentage of calories derived from fat in each serving. For more information on fat, see Chapter 4; for more information on sodium and salt, see Chapter 6; for more information on cholesterol, see Chapter 5.

BAGEL DANISH

1 Tbsp. Mock Cream Cheese (see recipe on page 220)
2 tsp. raisins
1 whole-wheat bagel, toasted
cinnamon

1. Spread Mock Cream Cheese and raisins on toasted bagel. Sprinkle with cinnamon.
2. Wrap in plastic wrap and microwave for 15–30 seconds until just warmed (or warm in regular oven, but then do not use plastic wrap).

Makes 1 serving. Each serving contains approximately 2 complex-carbohydrate exchanges, negligible dairy, negligible fat, 190 calories.

8% fat
199 mg sodium
1 mg cholesterol

BANANA FRENCH TOAST

1 banana
$\frac{1}{4}$ cup nonfat milk
1 tsp. vanilla extract
1 tsp. cinnamon
1 egg white
4 slices whole-wheat bread

1. Place all ingredients except bread into a blender and puree.
2. Pour mixture into a shallow soup bowl. Dip each slice of bread on both sides and place on a nonstick cookie sheet.
3. Bake for 15 minutes in a 350-degree oven, or grill on a nonstick grill. Serve immediately with fresh fruit preserves, sliced fruit, or fruit syrup.

Makes 4 servings. Each serving contains negligible dairy exchange, approximately $\frac{1}{4}$ fruit exchange, 1 complex-carbohydrate exchange, 100 calories.

7% fat
152 mg sodium
1 mg cholesterol

✗ BANANA ROLL-UP ✗

$\frac{1}{2}$ medium banana
1 Whole-Wheat Crepe (see p. 223)

3 oz. nonfat yogurt

Roll the banana in the crepe. Top it with the nonfat yogurt.

Makes 1 serving. Each serving contains approximately 1 fruit exchange, 1 complex-carbohydrate exchange, $\frac{1}{2}$ dairy exchange, 185 calories.

VARIATION:
Top with Fruit Syrup (see p. 267).

19% fat
22 mg sodium
1 mg cholesterol

✗ CHEESE BLINTZES ✗

Sauce
$\frac{2}{3}$ cup hoop cheese
$\frac{1}{2}$ cup nonfat buttermilk, or $\frac{1}{2}$ cup nonfat milk and $1\frac{1}{2}$ tsp. lemon juice

$\frac{1}{4}$ cup chopped fresh pineapple

Combine all the ingredients except pineapple in a blender container and blend until smooth. Pour the sauce into a bowl and add the pineapple.

Blintzes
2 cups hoop cheese
$\frac{1}{2}$ cup nonfat buttermilk, or $\frac{1}{2}$ cup nonfat milk and $1\frac{1}{2}$ tsp. lemon juice
2 Tbsp. apple juice concentrate

1 tsp. vanilla extract
1 tsp. ground cinnamon
1 medium banana
6 crepes* (see next recipe)

1. Combine all the ingredients except the crepes in a blender container and blend until smooth.

2. Spoon $\frac{1}{4}$ cup of mixture down the center of each crepe. Fold both sides of the crepe over toward the center. Place each crepe, seam side down, in a flat baking dish. Heat in a 350-degree oven until warm, about 10 minutes. Overcooking will toughen the crepe, and cheese filling mixture will harden and shrink.
3. To serve, place each blintz, seam side down, on a plate and spoon 2 Tbsp. of the sauce over the top of each. If desired, sprinkle with a little ground cinnamon for garnish.

Makes 6 blintzes. Each blintz contains approximately 1 dairy exchange, $\frac{1}{2}$ fruit exchange, 1 complex-carbohydrate exchange, 180 calories.

VARIATION:
TOPPING: Combine 1 cup nonfat yogurt, $\frac{1}{2}$ cup chopped fresh pineapple, 1 tsp. cinnamon, 1 tsp. vanilla extract, and $\frac{1}{4}$ cup nonfat milk. Serve chilled. Makes $1\frac{1}{3}$ cups. Each $\frac{1}{3}$ cup serving contains approximately $\frac{1}{4}$ dairy exchange, $\frac{1}{4}$ fruit exchange, 35 calories.

4% fat
66 mg sodium
4 mg cholesterol

✗ CREPES ✗

$\frac{2}{3}$ cup whole-wheat flour
2 Tbsp. rice flour
1 cup nonfat milk

1 tsp. apple juice concentrate
2 egg whites, stiffly beaten

1. Combine all ingredients except egg whites and mix thoroughly.
2. Fold stiffly beaten egg whites into mixture. Measure $\frac{1}{2}$ cup crepe batter per crepe and put onto a nonstick 8-inch crepe pan, tilting to cover inner surface of pan. Cook on both sides until golden brown.

NOTE: If you wish to make crepes ahead of time and freeze, place wax paper between them and wrap tightly so they are not exposed to air. Before using crepes, bring them to room temperature and heat until soft and pliable. If not reheated, they will break when folded.

Makes 6 crepes. Each crepe contains approximately 1 complex-carbohydrate exchange, negligible dairy exchange, 80 calories.

4% fat
56 mg sodium
1 mg cholesterol

✳ EGG ON A MUFFIN ✳

$\frac{1}{2}$ whole-wheat English muffin, toasted

2 egg whites, poached or hard-cooked

1 slice fresh tomato

1 sliced green chili (optional)

Top muffin with egg whites, tomato slice, and sliced green chili if desired.

Makes 1 serving. Each serving contains approximately 1 complex-carbohydrate exchange, $\frac{1}{2}$ vegetable exchange, 115 calories.

7% fat
116 mg sodium
0 mg cholesterol

✳ GRANOLA ✳

2 cups rolled oats

$\frac{1}{2}$ cup steel-cut oats

$1\frac{1}{2}$ cups wheat or rye flakes

$\frac{1}{2}$ cup rye flour or whole-wheat flour

$\frac{1}{4}$ cup powdered nonfat milk

$\frac{1}{2}$ cup millet

2 Tbsp. cinnamon

1 tsp. nutmeg

2 Tbsp. apple juice concentrate

2 tsp. vanilla

1 split vanilla bean

1. Place oats and wheat or rye flakes in a colander. Pour cold water over them just to dampen, then drain. Place in a bowl.
2. Add rye or whole-wheat flour, powdered milk, and millet. Mix gently with a fork and place on a nonstick baking sheet.
3. Sprinkle with half of cinnamon and nutmeg and with the combined apple juice concentrate and vanilla.
4. Toast in a 375-degree oven for 15 minutes. Add the remaining cinnamon and nutmeg. Mix lightly and toast for another 15 minutes. Repeat until the granola is golden brown—about 45 minutes total.
5. Cool and store in a tightly sealed jar to which you have added a split vanilla bean. Granola may be put into small plastic sandwich bags to be carried on trips, to the office, etc. It may be used as a cereal and topped with bananas, strawberries, blueberries, or peaches and cold milk.

Makes 6 cups. Each $\frac{1}{4}$ cup contains approximately 1 complex-carbohydrate exchange, 85 calories.

11% fat
52 mg sodium
1 mg cholesterol

✗ GRANOLA DATE BAR ✗

1 cup rolled oats
1 cup nugget cereal
1 cup crispy rice cereal
1 cup oat-bran flakes
1 Tbsp. cinnamon

$\frac{1}{2}$ tsp. nutmeg
1 cup dates, pitted and chopped
1 10-oz. jar no-sugar apricot
  preserves
3 egg whites, lightly beaten

1. Place dry ingredients in a bowl with the dates. Mix in the preserves. Mix in the egg whites.
2. Line a $15\frac{1}{2} \times 10\frac{1}{2}$–inch cookie tray (with sides) with parchment paper (available at kitchen-goods stores). Press mixture into tray. Bake for 15 minutes at 350 degrees. Remove from oven.
3. Lift the parchment paper with the partially baked mixture on it out of the tray and set it aside. Reline the tray with another piece of parchment paper. Invert the partially baked mixture onto the new paper. Remove the old paper and discard it.
4. Continue baking for another 15 minutes or until a light golden brown. Remove from oven. Cut into $1\frac{1}{2} \times 2$–inch bars while still warm.

Makes 50 bars. Each bar contains approximately $\frac{1}{2}$ complex-carbohydrate exchange, $\frac{1}{2}$ fruit exchange, 70 calories.

3% fat
27 mg sodium
0 mg cholesterol

✖ HOT NUGGET CEREAL ✖

2 Tbsp. nugget cereal
$\frac{1}{3}$ cup nonfat milk

1 Tbsp. apple juice concentrate

Mix all ingredients. Cover with plastic wrap and microwave for 2 to 3 minutes. Serve alone (or top with cold milk; milk will add 1 additional dairy exchange).

Makes 1 serving. Each serving contains approximately 1 complex-carbohydrate exchange, $\frac{1}{2}$ dairy exchange, $\frac{1}{2}$ fruit exchange, 155 calories.

2% fat
144 mg sodium
2 mg cholesterol

✖ HUEVOS RANCHEROS ✖

1 steamed corn tortilla
1 egg white, poached

$\frac{1}{4}$ cup green chilies
$\frac{1}{4}$ cup salsa

Top steamed tortilla with poached egg white, chiles, and salsa.

Makes 1 serving. Each serving contains approximately 1 complex-carbohydrate exchange, $\frac{1}{2}$ vegetable exchange, 93 calories.

VARIATION:
You may also add $\frac{1}{3}$ cup cooked beans (not refried) for 1 additional complex-carbohydrate exchange.

6% fat
156 mg sodium
0 mg cholesterol

✖ LATKES (POTATO PANCAKES) ✖

3 large potatoes, peeled and
　grated
Water to cover
$\frac{1}{2}$ cup grated onion
2 tsp. low-sodium soy sauce or
　tamari

1 tsp. Dijon-style mustard
$\frac{1}{4}$ tsp. baking powder
3 Tbsp. matzo meal
2 egg whites, stiffly beaten

1. Cover grated potatoes with water and let stand for 12 hours in refrigerator.
2. Drain well in strainer or colander and press out any excess moisture.
3. Add the grated onion to the potatoes and mix well.
4. Combine the soy sauce, mustard, baking powder, and matzo meal. Slowly add this to the potato mixture and mix thoroughly.
5. Fold in beaten egg whites and mix well.
6. Drop the mixture by tablespoonfuls onto a hot nonstick skillet. Cook until well browned on both sides.

Makes 16 latkes. Each latke contains approximately $\frac{1}{2}$ complex-carbohydrate exchange, negligible vegetable exchange, 45 calories.

VARIATIONS:
LATKES AND APPLESAUCE: Add $\frac{1}{4}$ cup unsweetened applesauce to each serving; adds $\frac{1}{2}$ fruit exchange and 20 calories per serving.

SALMON LATKES: Add 1 8-oz. can of water-packed salmon, drained and flaked, after Step 3, just before the matzo meal; adds $\frac{1}{2}$ protein exchange and 19 calories per serving.

2% fat
58 mg sodium
0 mg cholesterol

✖ MAPLE OATMEAL ✖

$\frac{1}{4}$ tsp. maple extract
1 cup hot cooked oatmeal

Add maple extract to oatmeal while cooking.

Makes 1 serving. Each serving contains approximately 2 complex-carbohydrate exchanges, 150 calories.

14% fat
2 mg sodium
0 mg cholesterol

✖ MEXICAN EGGS ✖

$\frac{1}{4}$ cup diced onions
2 Tbsp. diced red bell peppers
2 Tbsp. diced green bell peppers
1 recipe Scrambled Eggs à la
   Longevity (see p. 222)

1 Tbsp. green chili salsa (or
   more, to taste)

1. Steam the vegetables until they are crisp and tender, for about 5 minutes.
2. Prepare Scrambled Eggs à la Longevity, cooking to desired degree.
3. Add vegetables and salsa. Cook for 1 minute more.

NOTE: Do not add steamed vegetable mix to uncooked eggs. Cook eggs first.

Makes 4 servings. Each serving contains approximately $\frac{1}{4}$ dairy exchange, $\frac{1}{4}$ vegetable exchange, 60 calories.

1% fat
139 mg sodium
1 mg cholesterol

✄ MOCK CREAM CHEESE ✄

1 pound fresh hoop cheese   Up to $\frac{1}{2}$ cup nonfat milk

1. Crumble the hoop cheese into a food processor. Process until it forms a ball.
2. Add the milk gradually while creaming the cheese. When the mixture is smooth, store covered in the refrigerator.

NOTE: This cream-cheese mixture may be frozen. However, it forms ice crystals which must be beaten out before using.

Makes 2 cups. Each 1-Tbsp. serving contains negligible dairy exchange, approximately 25 calories.

VARIATION:
MOCK SOUR CREAM: Use buttermilk instead of milk, or add 1 tsp. lemon juice or vinegar. Add gradually to the hoop cheese until desired sour-cream consistency is achieved.

9% fat
6 mg sodium
1 mg cholesterol

✄ OAT-BRAN MUFFINS ✄

$2\frac{1}{4}$ cups oat bran
$1\frac{1}{4}$ Tbsp. cinnamon
1 Tbsp. low-sodium baking powder
$\frac{1}{2}$ cup nonfat milk
$\frac{3}{4}$ cup apple juice concentrate

1 medium apple, cored and grated
$\frac{1}{4}$ cup raisins
2 egg whites
Nonstick cooking spray

1. Mix dry ingredients in a large bowl.
2. In a separate bowl, mix the milk, apple juice concentrate, apple, and raisins; add to dry ingredients and mix.

3. Beat egg whites until foamy. Fold into batter.
4. Spray muffin pans with nonstick cooking spray; wipe off excess.
5. Bake at 350 degrees for 17 minutes. When cool, store in a plastic bag to retain softness and moisture.

Makes 12 muffins (12 servings). Each serving contains approximately 1 complex-carbohydrate exchange, ½ fruit exchange, 120 calories.

13% fat
20 mg sodium
0 mg cholesterol

OATMEAL PANCAKES

¼ cup rolled oats
¼ cup nonfat buttermilk
½ tsp. baking soda, or 1 tsp. low-sodium baking powder
¼ cup whole-wheat pastry flour
2 tsp. apple juice concentrate
½ tsp. vanilla
1 egg white

1. Chop the rolled oats coarsely in a blender or food processor.
2. Add buttermilk to the rolled oats, combine, and let stand for a few minutes.
3. Add all the other ingredients to the blender container and blend until well mixed.
4. Cook on a nonstick griddle or skillet using ¼ cup batter for each pancake.

NOTE: Serve with chopped fresh strawberries and bananas or whatever other fresh fruit is available, or Fruit Syrup (see p. 267; these fruit additions would add 1 fruit exchange).

Makes six 6-inch pancakes. Each pancake contains approximately 1 complex-carbohydrate exchange, 80 calories.

7% fat
14 mg sodium
0 mg cholesterol

PEACH OATMEAL

½ cup hot cooked oatmeal
1½ Tbsp. Pritikin brand peach fruit spread

Top cooked oatmeal with peach fruit spread. Stir to mix if desired.

Makes 1 serving. Each serving contains approximately 1 complex-carbohydrate exchange, 1 fruit exchange, 140 calories.

8% fat
1 mg sodium
0 mg cholesterol

SCRAMBLED EGGS À LA LONGEVITY

1 cup egg whites (8 egg whites)
3 Tbsp. liquid nonfat milk
3 Tbsp. powdered nonfat milk
¼ tsp. onion powder
½ tsp. cornstarch
Pinch turmeric
¼ tsp. low-sodium tamari
Nonstick cooking spray (optional)

1. Blend the egg whites and liquid milk together until well mixed.
2. Thoroughly mix together the remaining dry ingredients. Add these to the milk/egg mixture along with the tamari, mixing well.
3. Using a nonstick skillet or pan or a double boiler coated with nonstick cooking spray, cook as you would other scrambled eggs, stirring frequently.

Makes 4 servings. Each serving contains negligible dairy exchange, negligible vegetable exchange, approximately 60 calories.

1% fat
139 mg sodium
1 mg cholesterol

✖ WHOLE-WHEAT CREPES ✖

1 cup sifted whole-wheat flour, or 1 cup whole-wheat pastry flour
1 cup nonfat milk
$\frac{1}{4}$ cup mineral water (add more if batter is too thick)

1 tsp. frozen apple juice concentrate
$\frac{1}{2}$ cup egg whites (4–5 egg whites)
$\frac{1}{4}$ tsp. freshly grated nutmeg
Nonstick cooking spray

1. Place flour in a blender or food processor. Add milk, mineral water, frozen apple juice concentrate, egg whites, and nutmeg. Blend until smooth and has the consistency of heavy cream.
2. Cover and store in refrigerator until cold.
3. Heat a 7-inch seasoned nonstick crepe pan. (Spray with nonstick cooking spray before heating and as needed.) Pour $\frac{1}{4}$ cup of the batter at a time into the pan. Tilt from side to side to spread the batter evenly. Cook over medium heat until the edges start to curl, then carefully turn the crepe with a spatula and brown the other side. Repeat until all of the batter is used. To keep the crepes pliable, put them in a covered casserole in a warm oven.

NOTE: To freeze the crepes, put a piece of waxed paper between each crepe and wrap them well so that they are not exposed to air. Before using, bring to room temperature and put in a preheated 300-degree oven for 20 minutes or until soft and pliable. If not reheated, crepes will break when folded.

Makes 8 crepes. Each crepe contains approximately 1 complex-carbohydrate exchange, negligible dairy exchange, 70 calories.

SUGGESTED FILLINGS: Stir-"fried" vegetables, mushrooms, hoop cheese.

VARIATIONS:
SPINACH CREPE: Add $\frac{1}{3}$ cup frozen chopped spinach (defrosted and wrung out) and 1 tsp. chopped onion to the basic recipe. Since spinach may thicken the mixture, it may be necessary to add up to $\frac{1}{4}$ cup more water.

4% fat
39 mg sodium
1 mg cholesterol

ENTREES

✖ ARTICHOKE PÂTÉ ✖

2 cups hoop cheese
$\frac{1}{2}$ cup chopped onion
2 tsp. garlic powder
1 cup chopped artichoke hearts,
  drained, rinsed

1 cup chopped asparagus,
  blanched, or 1 cup chopped
  spinach, drained
Lettuce leaves
Garnish

1. Combine first five ingredients in a food processor. Blend until creamy.
2. Line a mold with plastic wrap. Put mixture in mold and chill for 30 minutes. Unmold on lettuce leaves. Garnish as desired.

NOTE: When using spinach, add $\frac{1}{2}$ tsp. or more of Italian seasoning.

Makes 9 servings. Each $\frac{1}{2}$-cup serving contains approximately $\frac{1}{2}$ dairy exchange, negligible vegetable exchange, 50 calories.

7% fat
15 mg sodium
0 mg cholesterol

CANNELLONI

- 1⅓ cups hoop cheese
- ½ cup nonfat milk
- ½ tsp. oregano, crushed
- ¼ tsp. nutmeg
- ½ tsp. basil, crushed
- 2 egg whites, stiffly beaten
- 3 cups Marinara Sauce (see p. 268)
- 6 Crepes (see p. 214)

1. Put hoop cheese, milk, oregano, nutmeg, and basil in a blender container and blend until smooth.
2. Spoon blended hoop cheese into a bowl and fold in the beaten egg whites.
3. Cover the bottom of a 9 × 9–inch baking dish with half of the Marinara Sauce.
4. Divide cheese mixture evenly down the centers of the crepes. Fold crepes over and place, seam side down, in the baking dish.
5. Bake at 375 degrees for 10 to 15 minutes or until hot. Do not overheat or the cheese will harden and shrink. Spoon the remaining sauce over the top of the cannelloni before serving.

Makes 6 cannelloni. Each cannelloni contains approximately ¾ dairy exchange, 2 vegetable exchanges, 1 complex-carbohydrate exchange, 185 calories.

5% fat
93 mg sodium
1 mg cholesterol

CHICKEN À L'ORANGE

- 1 tsp. prepared mustard
- ¼ cup orange marmalade (no sugar or honey added)
- ¼ to ½ cup wine
- ½ cup sliced onion
- 2 chicken breasts (4 to 4½ oz. each), cut in julienne strips

Combine mustard, marmalade, and wine in a skillet. Add onion and chicken. Simmer for about 5 to 8 minutes or until done as desired.

NOTE: Serve over rice, pasta, or any grain of choice.

Makes 2 servings. Each serving contains negligible fruit exchange, negligible vegetable exchange, approximately $3\frac{1}{2}$ oz. high protein, 240 calories.

17% fat   90 mg cholesterol
100 mg sodium

✕ CHICKEN CURRY ✕

1	cup unpeeled chopped apple	$\frac{2}{3}$	cup instant nonfat milk powder
1	cup sliced celery		
$\frac{1}{2}$	cup chopped onion	1 to 2	tsp. curry powder (to taste)
1	clove garlic, minced		
2	Tbsp. plus $1\frac{1}{2}$ cups defatted chicken stock	2	Tbsp. cornstarch
		2	cups diced cooked chicken (12 oz.)
1	cup sliced mushrooms		
		$\frac{1}{2}$	cup fresh or frozen peas, cooked

1. In a saucepan, combine apple, celery, onion, and garlic in 2 Tbsp. chicken stock. Cook until the onion is translucent. Add the mushrooms and cook for 2 minutes longer.
2. Combine the remaining chicken stock, nonfat milk powder, curry powder, and cornstarch. Stir into vegetable mixture. Cook and stir until mixture thickens and bubbles.
3. Add the chicken and peas. Heat through.

NOTE: Serve with brown rice and various condiments such as raisins, sliced green onion, chopped red apple, grated egg white, and chopped tomatoes.

Makes 4 servings. Each 1-cup serving contains approximately $\frac{1}{2}$ dairy exchange, negligible fruit, vegetable, and complex-carbohydrate exchanges, 3 oz. high protein, 275 calories.

VARIATION:
Substitute 12 oz. raw chicken for the cooked chicken. "Sauté" first with some of the chicken stock.

15% fat   72 mg cholesterol
308 mg sodium

✖ CHICKEN IN RASPBERRY MARINADE ✖

8	4-oz. chicken breasts, boned		Dash hot pepper sauce
1	Tbsp. low-sodium soy sauce	2	cloves garlic
3 oz.	pineapple juice concentrate	$1\frac{1}{2}$	tsp. powdered ginger
$\frac{1}{8}$	tsp. chili powder	4 oz.	pureed raspberry preserves, unsweetened
$\frac{1}{8}$	tsp. sweet basil	1	Tbsp. rice vinegar
$\frac{1}{8}$	tsp. curry powder	1	Tbsp. crushed, dried red peppers
			Water to cover

1. Remove the skin from the chicken.
2. Combine the remaining ingredients. Pour them over the chicken in a shallow dish and marinate overnight.
3. Grill the chicken, brushing occasionally with the marinade, or put a small amount of marinade in a pan and bake the chicken until done, about 20–25 minutes.
4. Freeze any remaining marinade for later use.

Makes 8 servings. Each serving contains approximately $\frac{1}{2}$ fruit exchange, $3\frac{1}{2}$ oz. high protein, 200 calories.

15% fat   78 mg cholesterol
110 mg sodium

CRANBERRY-GLAZED CHICKEN BREAST WITH ✖ WHOLE-GRAIN STUFFING ✖

4	chicken breast halves, boned and skinned	$\frac{1}{2}$ cup cranberry preserves, with no added sugar
1	cup cooked whole-grain cereal (cooked in chicken broth)	$\frac{1}{2}$ tsp. low-sodium soy sauce
$\frac{1}{4}$	cup unsweetened cranberry juice concentrate	$\frac{1}{2}$ tsp. low-sodium Dijon mustard
		$\frac{1}{3}$ cup dry white wine

1. With a sharp knife, slice each chicken breast in half horizontally, but not quite all the way through, to form a pocket. Stuff the chicken breast pockets with the cooked grain cereal and place them in an ovenproof baking dish.
2. Combine the cranberry juice concentrate, cranberry preserves, soy

sauce, Dijon mustard, and dry white wine in a bowl, and whisk together until thoroughly mixed.
3. Pour two-thirds of the sauce over the chicken breasts and bake uncovered in a preheated 350-degree oven for 30 minutes, basting occasionally.
4. Heat the remaining sauce. Serve the chicken breasts topped with 1 tablespoon of the hot cranberry sauce.

NOTE: For a more interesting stuffing, cook the grain cereal in chicken broth with $\frac{1}{2}$ small chopped onion and $\frac{1}{2}$ cup sliced mushrooms.

Makes 4 servings. Each serving contains approximately 1 fruit exchange, 1 complex-carbohydrate exchange, $3\frac{1}{2}$ oz. high protein, 330 calories.

10% fat   84 mg cholesterol
207 mg sodium

✖ FISH IN LIME SAUCE ✖

1 pound orange roughy, sea   3 limes
  bass, sole, or other delicate fish   5 small sprigs fresh dill
$\frac{1}{2}$ cup unsweetened pineapple
  juice

1. Cut fish into four 4-oz. fillets. Place in nonstick baking dish with pineapple juice.
2. Grate peel of one lime and add to pan. Squeeze juice from all limes and add to pan with one sprig of dill.
3. Cook covered at 350 degrees. Fish requires 8 minutes of cooking per $\frac{1}{2}$ inch of thickness.
4. Remove cooked sprig of dill. Put fish on a platter. Top with pan juices and garnish each fillet with a sprig of dill or additional slices of lime.

NOTE: Fish fillets can also be cooked on stovetop. Use a nonstick skillet and cook, covered, over medium heat until fillets flake when lightly touched, about 8 minutes per $\frac{1}{2}$ inch thickness.

Makes 4 servings. Each serving contains negligible fruit exchange, approximately 3 oz. high protein, 175 calories.

40% fat   23 mg cholesterol
73 mg sodium

✖ MINI MEATBALLS ✖

8 oz.	ground turkey breast	$\frac{1}{4}$	cup chopped parsley
1	cup prepared bulgur wheat	1 or 2	egg whites
		1	tsp. poultry seasoning

1. Combine all the ingredients in a bowl.
2. Take a small amount of mixture and roll it into a ball. Place it on a cookie sheet. Make 16 meatballs.
3. Bake in a 350-degree oven for 10 to 15 minutes or until all are cooked through and lightly browned.

Makes 4 servings. Each serving contains approximately $\frac{1}{2}$ complex-carbohydrate exchange, 2 oz. high protein, 120 calories.

20% fat   40 mg cholesterol
66 mg sodium

✖ ORIENTAL RICE ✖

2 tsp. minced ginger	1 cup diced bell pepper
2 large cloves garlic, minced	1 cup diced carrots
$\frac{1}{2}$ cup defatted chicken stock	1 cup sliced water chestnuts
3 Tbsp. reduced-sodium soy sauce	4 cups cooked brown rice
	1 cup chopped green onions
3 cups sliced mushrooms	$1\frac{1}{2}$ tsp. sesame seeds, toasted
2 cups sliced bok choy	

1. "Sauté" ginger and garlic in $\frac{1}{4}$ cup chicken stock and soy sauce.
2. Add mushrooms, bok choy, bell pepper, carrots, water chestnuts, and rice. Cook until vegetables are tender, adding more chicken stock as needed.
3. Add green onion and sesame seeds.

Makes 10 servings. Each 1-cup serving contains approximately 1 complex-carbohydrate exchange, 1 vegetable exchange, 120 calories.

7% fat   0 mg cholesterol
173 mg sodium

✖ PINEAPPLE CHICKEN ✖

1	tsp. fresh grated ginger	$\frac{1}{4}$	tsp. poultry seasoning
1	garlic clove, minced	$\frac{3}{4}$	cup sliced red and green
1	shallot, minced		peppers
1	cup defatted chicken stock	1	cup cubed fresh pineapple
$\frac{3}{4}$	cup chopped onions	$\frac{1}{4}$	cup tomato puree
6 oz.	pineapple juice	1	Tbsp. cornstarch
9 oz.	boneless, skinless, cooked	$\frac{1}{4}$	cup water
	chicken breasts, cubed	1	Tbsp. apple juice concentrate
1	Tbsp. low-sodium soy		
	sauce		

1. Put ginger, garlic, and shallot in a large saucepan with the chicken stock and simmer for 10 minutes.
2. Add the onion and cook for 5 minutes. Add the pineapple juice. Simmer for 1 minute.
3. Add chicken, soy sauce, seasoning, peppers, pineapple, and tomato puree. Simmer for 10 minutes.
4. Dissolve cornstarch in water and apple juice concentrate. Blend into chicken mixture. Simmer, stirring constantly, until thickened and clear. Cook for 1 minute more.

NOTE: Serve over brown rice or other grain.

Makes 3 servings. Each serving contains approximately 1 fruit exchange, 1 vegetable exchange, 3 oz. high protein, 240 calories.

10% fat
198 mg sodium
80 mg cholesterol

✖ PITA-BREAD PIZZA ✖

4 sandwich-size pita breads
   (about 4 inches in diameter)
2 cups tomato sauce, or Pritikin
   brand spaghetti sauce
$\frac{1}{2}$ tsp. Italian seasoning
1 medium zucchini, shredded

1 small onion, thinly sliced
$\frac{1}{2}$ cup sliced mushrooms
$\frac{1}{2}$ cup diced or sliced bell pepper
$\frac{1}{2}$ cup crumbled nonfat cottage
   cheese or hoop cheese
Sapsago cheese, grated, to taste

1. Separate pita bread into halves. Place on a nonstick baking sheet, smooth side down, and bake for 5 minutes at 400 degrees or until crisp.
2. Combine the tomato sauce and Italian seasoning. Spread this mixture on the pita halves using $1\frac{1}{2}$ Tbsp. per half. Top with the vegetables, dividing evenly.
3. Sprinkle each pizza with 1 Tbsp. of the nonfat cheese. Sprinkle each with the grated Sapsago cheese.
4. Bake at 350 degrees until hot, approximately 10 minutes.

NOTE: To separate the pita bread easily, place in a microwave oven for 10 to 15 seconds to soften.

Makes 8 pizzas. Each pizza contains approximately $\frac{1}{2}$ dairy exchange, 1 complex-carbohydrate exchange, 2 vegetable exchanges, 160 calories.

6% fat
17 mg sodium
1 mg cholesterol

RATATOUILLE

1 medium eggplant
6 medium zucchini
2 green bell peppers
2 large onions, sliced
4 large tomatoes, cut into chunks
1 clove garlic, minced
½ cup minced parsley
1 tsp. crushed oregano
1 tsp. low-sodium soy sauce

1. Cut unpeeled eggplant into ½-inch cubes. Slice zucchini into ½-inch rounds. Remove seeds from green bell peppers and cut into ½-inch squares.
2. Combine all ingredients and mix thoroughly.
3. Place mixture in a 6-quart casserole with a cover. Bake at 350 degrees for 1½ hours, covered, and ½ hour uncovered. During the first hour, baste top occasionally with some of the liquid to ensure even flavoring.
4. Serve hot from the oven, or cold. Cool to room temperature before refrigerating. Flavors are enhanced if chilled and then reheated before serving.

Makes 8 servings. Each serving contains approximately 3 vegetable exchanges, 75 calories.

VARIATION:
Place all ingredients in a 6-quart pot. Add ½ cup red wine, ½ cup tomato juice. Cook covered on top of stove for 35 minutes.

8% fat
33 mg sodium
0 mg cholesterol

✗ RED SNAPPER VERACRUZ ✗

Sauce

2 tomatoes, peeled and diced
1 large onion, peeled and
  coarsely chopped
1 small jalapeño pepper,
  chopped fine (use gloves!)

3 Tbsp. capers, rinsed
Juice of 2 limes
2 cloves garlic, minced
$\frac{1}{4}$ cup water

Combine the above ingredients and simmer for 15 minutes.

Fish

4 4-oz. red snapper fillets
1 sprig cilantro

Simmer the fish in the sauce for approximately 10 minutes, or until the fish is opaque. Chop the cilantro and sprinkle it over the top of the fish.

Makes 4 servings. Each serving contains approximately 1 vegetable exchange, 3 oz. high protein, 130 calories.

10% fat
331 mg sodium
42 mg cholesterol

✗ SALMON PÂTÉ ✗

$\frac{1}{3}$ cup hoop cheese
1 15$\frac{1}{2}$-oz. can red salmon
3 artichoke hearts, rinsed and
  drained
1 green onion
3 Tbsp. chopped fresh dill, or 1
  Tbsp. dried crushed dill weed

6 drops hot pepper sauce
1 tsp. salt-free Dijon mustard
1 Tbsp. freshly squeezed
   lemon juice
1 Tbsp. capers, rinsed and
   drained
2 oz. pimentos, drained

1. Blend hoop cheese (alone) in a blender or food processor into a ball of fine, smooth texture first (necessary for a pâté of smooth consistency).
2. Place the salmon in the blender or food processor with the hoop

cheese; add artichokes, green onion, fresh dill, hot pepper sauce, mustard, lemon juice, and capers and blend well. Add pimentos and blend, leaving specks visible.

3. Chill for several hours or overnight to permit the flavors to blend.

NOTE: Serve chilled with raw vegetables or crackers. Garnish with cucumber and fresh chopped dill if desired.

Makes $2\frac{1}{2}$ cups (10–12 servings, $\frac{1}{4}$ cup each, as an appetizer). Each appetizer serving contains approximately $1\frac{1}{2}$ oz. high protein, negligible dairy exchange, negligible vegetable exchange, 80 calories.

38% fat
74 mg sodium
20 mg cholesterol

✕ SCALLOPED POTATOES ✕

1 cup finely chopped onion
$1\frac{1}{2}$ cups defatted chicken stock
$1\frac{1}{4}$ cups powdered nonfat milk
2 Tbsp. cornstarch

1 Tbsp. low-sodium soy sauce
$\frac{1}{2}$ tsp. unsalted prepared mustard
4 cups thinly sliced potatoes

1. "Sauté" onion in a little of the chicken stock. Combine all the other ingredients except the potatoes with the remaining chicken stock and mix well.
2. Place one layer of potatoes in a nonstick baking pan and cover with the onions. Then follow with another layer of potatoes.
3. Pour the chicken-stock mixture over the potatoes. There should be just enough to cover them. Cover the pan with foil. Bake at 300 degrees until potatoes are done, about 1 hour.

Makes 6 servings. Each $\frac{2}{3}$-cup serving contains approximately $\frac{1}{2}$ dairy exchange, 1 complex-carbohydrate exchange, 140 calories.

2% fat
271 mg sodium
5 mg cholesterol

✖ SPICY BEEF ✖

Spicy Beef

8 oz.	flank steak, cut across the grain into bite-size servings
3	Tbsp. sherry
1	clove garlic, crushed
1	large onion, coarsely chopped
1	large green pepper, diced
1	large red pepper, diced

3	stalks celery, cut into diagonal slices
3	stalks bok choy, cut into diagonal slices
1	8-oz. can water chestnuts, drained and sliced
3	green onions, sliced (use green tops also)

Marinade (mix these together)

2 Tbsp. low-sodium soy sauce
1 Tbsp. apple juice concentrate
3 tsp. chili powder

$\frac{1}{8}$ tsp. ginger powder
$\frac{1}{4}$ tsp. garlic powder
Dash cayenne pepper

Sauce (mix these together)

1 tsp. apple juice concentrate
$\frac{1}{2}$ tsp. curry powder
1 Tbsp. low-sodium soy sauce (dilute if necessary)

1 tsp. cornstarch
3 Tbsp. water

1. Prepare the marinade and the sauce. Marinate the beef for 30 minutes or longer in the marinade.
2. Heat the sherry and crushed garlic in a wok (or skillet). "Sauté" the marinated beef in the sherry and add any remaining marinade to the wok. Remove the meat to a platter (leave the liquid).
3. Stir-"fry" the vegetables, adding each at 1-minute intervals in the following order: onion, green pepper, red pepper, celery, bok choy, water chestnuts, and green onions.
4. Add sauce and cook, stirring until thickened.
5. Mix in meat and cook until well heated.

NOTE: Serve over rice or noodles.

Makes 6 servings. Each serving contains approximately $1\frac{1}{2}$ oz. high protein, 3 vegetable exchanges, 160 calories.

VARIATION:
Substitute tofu, cut into bite-size pieces, for beef.

35% fat
26 mg cholesterol
314 mg sodium

TERIYAKI CHICKEN

2 whole chicken breasts (approx. 8 oz. each), boned, skinned, and halved
1 cup Teriyaki Marinade (see next recipe)
2 medium onions, thinly sliced
1 16-oz. can pineapple slices, packed in their natural juice, undrained
1 Tbsp. cornstarch

1. Marinate chicken breasts in Teriyaki Marinade for at least 2 hours before cooking. Preheat oven to 350 degrees.
2. "Sauté" onions until tender and lightly browned. Spoon half of the onions into a shallow baking dish. Remove the chicken breasts from the marinade and set the marinade aside. Arrange the chicken breasts on top of the onions. Do no overlap the pieces. Place the remaining onions evenly over the top of the chicken.
3. Remove the pineapple slices from the can, saving the juice. Arrange the pineapple slices evenly over the top of the onions in the baking dish. Cover the dish and bake for 25 to 30 minutes, or until done.
4. Pour the pineapple juice into a saucepan. Add 2 Tbsp. of the marinade to it. Add the cornstarch and mix thoroughly until the cornstarch is dissolved. Bring the pineapple juice mixture to a boil and simmer, stirring constantly, until slightly thickened.
5. Remove the chicken from the oven and pour the pineapple sauce evenly over the top. Serve each piece of chicken with 2 pineapple rings on top.

Makes 4 servings. Each serving contains approximately 1 fruit exchange, 1 vegetable exchange, 3½ oz. high protein, 350 calories.

VARIATION:
Substitute ½ pound of flank steak for the chicken.

8% fat
87 mg cholesterol
143 mg sodium

✖ TERIYAKI MARINADE ✖

$\frac{1}{3}$ cup low-sodium soy sauce
$\frac{2}{3}$ cup water
2 Tbsp. apple juice concentrate

2 cloves garlic, crushed
$1\frac{1}{2}$ tsp. freshly grated ginger root, or $\frac{1}{4}$ tsp. ground ginger

Combine all the ingredients and mix well. Store in the refrigerator. (For best results, make marinade at least 24 hours in advance.)

Makes about 1 cup. Each cup contains approximately 1 fruit exchange; calories per serving are negligible when used only as a marinade (meat absorbs approximately $\frac{1}{4}$ of the marinade).

VARIATIONS:
When used with:

BEEF:
Add another 2 Tbsp. apple juice concentrate (60 calories).

CHICKEN:
Add 2 Tbsp. pineapple juice concentrate (64 calories).

FISH:
Reduce the water to $\frac{1}{3}$ cup and add $\frac{1}{2}$ cup sherry (107 calories).

1% fat
917 mg sodium
0 mg cholesterol

✗ TERIYAKI STEAK ✗

1 pound round steak
1 cup Teriyaki Marinade (see
  preceding recipe)

1. Remove all visible fat from round steak.
2. Pour marinade over steak and allow to marinate for at least 2 hours before cooking.
3. Remove steak from marinade and place on a broiler pan. Place under broiler and cook for 2 to 3 minutes per side for rare steak. Cook longer if desired.

Makes 4 servings. Each serving contains approximately 3 oz. high protein, 200 calories.

VARIATION:
Substitute chicken breasts for round steak.

30% fat
140 mg sodium
78 mg cholesterol

✖ VEGETARIAN MOO SHOO ✖

Glaze

$\frac{1}{3}$ cup defatted chicken stock

1 Tbsp. apple juice concentrate
    or pineapple juice concentrate

1 Tbsp. low-sodium soy sauce or
    tamari

3 Tbsp. cornstarch

Combine all glaze ingredients and set aside.

Stir-Fry

2 large garlic cloves, minced

1 Tbsp. minced fresh ginger root

1 cup defatted chicken stock

1 cup celery, sliced Chinese style
    (cut on the diagonal)

1 cup pea pods

1 cup sliced onion ($\frac{1}{2}$-inch slices)

$\frac{1}{2}$ green pepper, diced

$\frac{1}{2}$ red pepper, diced

$\frac{1}{2}$ cup bok choy, sliced Chinese
    style

$\frac{1}{2}$ cup finely chopped Napa
    cabbage

1 cup sliced mushrooms

6 stalks asparagus, or 6 stalks
    broccoli, sliced Chinese style

$\frac{1}{2}$ cup sliced water chestnuts

6 Whole-Wheat Crepes with
    spinach variation, warm (see
    p. 223)

Chopped parsley

1. Cook garlic and ginger in chicken stock. Add celery and pea pods and cook for 2 minutes. Add onion, green pepper, red pepper, and bok choy and cook for 2 minutes. Add Napa, mushrooms, asparagus (or broccoli), and water chestnuts and cook until vegetables are tender yet crisp.
2. Add glaze mixture to vegetables and cook until glaze becomes transparent and shiny.
3. Spoon mixture down the center of each crepe. Fold both sides of crepe over toward the center. Place crepes, seam side down, in a glass or nonstick pan.
4. Bake uncovered for 15 minutes at 375 degrees. Garnish with chopped parsley and serve.

NOTE: To add color and variety, add 2 or 3 carrots and 1 or 2 crookneck squash cut into matchstick shapes.

Makes 6 servings. Each serving contains approximately 1 complex-carbohydrate exchange, 2 vegetable exchanges, 125 calories.

VARIATION:
Omit crepes. Serve as stir-fry over brown rice. Makes 6 servings. Each serving (without the rice) contains approximately $\frac{1}{4}$ complex-carbohydrate exchange, $2\frac{1}{4}$ vegetable exchanges, 72 calories.

4% fat
150 mg sodium
1 mg cholesterol

SOUPS

✗ BLACK-BEAN SOUP ✗

2	cups black beans	$\frac{3}{4}$	cup red wine
6–8	cups water	2	Tbsp. red wine vinegar
$1\frac{1}{2}$	medium onions, chopped	$\frac{1}{2}$	tsp. dried thyme
1	large clove garlic, minced	$\frac{1}{2}$	tsp. dried oregano
$1\frac{1}{2}$	cups chopped tomatoes	2	Tbsp. low-sodium soy sauce
1	cup chopped celery	$\frac{3}{4}$	cup nonfat yogurt
2	cups chopped green pepper	$\frac{3}{4}$	cup chopped green onion
1	jalapeño pepper, diced (use gloves!)	$1\frac{1}{2}$	Tbsp. chopped cilantro

1. Soak the beans according to package directions
2. Cook the beans in the water with the onion and garlic for $1\frac{1}{2}$ to 2 hours, until tender.
3. Add the tomato, celery, green pepper, jalapeño pepper, red wine, red wine vinegar, thyme, oregano, and soy sauce. Continue cooking for 1 hour or more.
4. Serve with garnish of 1 Tbsp. of yogurt, 1 Tbsp. of chopped green onion, and a sprinkle of cilantro (or 1 Tbsp. of salsa).

Makes 10 cups. Each 1-cup serving contains approximately 1 complex-carbohydrate exchange, 1 vegetable exchange, negligible dairy exchange, 130 calories.

4% fat
128 mg sodium
1 mg cholesterol

✖ CHINESE TOMATO SOUP ✖

1 green chili, seeded, rinsed, and
　finely chopped
$\frac{1}{2}$ cup salt-free tomato sauce
1 15-oz. can unsalted tomatoes
3 cups water
1 cup diagonally cut bok choy
1 stalk celery without leaves,
　thinly sliced

1 medium onion, thinly sliced
2 cloves garlic, minced
1 cup bean sprouts
$\frac{1}{2}$ cup chopped green onion
$\frac{1}{4}$ cup cooked brown rice
1 Tbsp. low-sodium soy sauce
$\frac{1}{2}$ tsp. curry powder
Dash chili powder

1. Combine the chili, tomato sauce, tomatoes, water, bok choy, celery, onion, and garlic. Cook for about 15 minutes.
2. Add bean sprouts, green onion, rice, soy sauce, curry powder, and chili powder and mix thoroughly. Turn off heat and let soup sit for 10 minutes before serving.

Makes 6 servings. Each 1-cup serving contains approximately 2 vegetable exchanges, 50 calories.

3% fat
74 mg sodium

0 mg cholesterol

✖ COLD CUCUMBER SOUP ✖

4 cucumbers or 2 large hothouse
　cucumbers, peeled and cut into
　chunks
3 green onions
$\frac{1}{2}$ cup fresh parsley
2 cloves garlic
3 Tbsp. chopped fresh dill, or 1
　Tbsp. crushed dried dill weed

1　　quart nonfat buttermilk
1　　Tbsp. freshly squeezed
　　　lemon juice
4 to 6 drops hot pepper sauce
Cucumber slices for garnish
Mock Sour Cream for garnish
　(see p. 268)

1. Combine all ingredients except lemon juice and hot pepper sauce in a blender container. Blend until smooth.
2. Add lemon juice and hot pepper sauce and mix well.
3. Chill 4 to 6 hours before serving. Serve in chilled bowls garnished with cucumber slices and Mock Sour Cream.

NOTE: If Mock Sour Cream is used, add $\frac{1}{4}$ dairy exchange and 25 calories per 2 Tbsp.

Makes 8 1-cup servings. Each serving contains approximately $\frac{1}{2}$ dairy exchange, $\frac{1}{2}$ vegetable exchange, 60 calories.

22% fat   3 mg cholesterol
49 mg sodium

✖ GAZPACHO ✖

4 large ripe tomatoes, peeled and seeded
1 large cucumber, peeled and seeded, or $\frac{1}{2}$ Belgian or European cucumber (no peeling or seeding required)
1 bell pepper
$\frac{1}{2}$ small red or white onion
2 shallots
1 large clove garlic

1 10-oz. can low-sodium tomato juice
1 cup defatted chicken stock
6 drops hot pepper sauce
$\frac{1}{2}$ cup red wine vinegar
1 tsp. paprika
1 Tbsp. fresh oregano, or 1 tsp. crushed dried oregano
Garnish vegetables or croutons (see Step 2)

1. Puree tomatoes, cucumber, pepper, onion, shallots, and garlic. Place in a bowl and add tomato juice, chicken stock, hot pepper sauce, vinegar, paprika, and oregano. Blend thoroughly.
2. Chill several hours before serving. Serve with the following diced vegetables as a garnish: green pepper, red pepper, cucumber, green onion, or peeled, seeded tomato. Or sprinkle with garlic croutons made from Pritikin brand bread and fresh garlic.

Makes 5 servings. Each 1-cup serving contains approximately 2 vegetable exchanges, 50 calories.

VARIATION:
May also be served with Mock Sour Cream (see p. 268) and freshly chopped dill.

6% fat   0 mg cholesterol
57 mg sodium

✖ SHERRIED PEA SOUP ✖

2 cups fresh peas
1 cup defatted chicken stock
2 Tbsp. sherry

Dash cayenne pepper
1 cup nonfat milk
$\frac{1}{2}$ tsp. grated lemon peel

1. Combine the peas, chicken stock, sherry, and cayenne pepper in a saucepan. Bring to a boil, cover, and cook until the peas are tender, about 5 minutes.
2. Cool slightly and pour the peas and their liquid into a blender container. Add the milk and blend until smooth.
3. Pour the soup into a container, cover, and refrigerate until cold.
4. Pour the cold soup into chilled bowls. Sprinkle each serving with a pinch of grated lemon peel.

NOTE: This soup may be frozen.

Makes 4 servings. Each 1-cup serving contains approximately $\frac{1}{4}$ dairy exchange, 1 complex-carbohydrate exchange, 90 calories.

VARIATION:
Add up to $1\frac{3}{4}$ oz. per serving of cooked shredded crabmeat. Each 1 oz. adds 1 protein exchange and 37 calories.

6% fat
37 mg sodium
1 mg cholesterol

SALADS AND SALAD DRESSINGS

✗ CARROT SALAD ✗

6 cups grated carrots
$\frac{1}{4}$ cup freshly squeezed lemon
juice

$\frac{1}{4}$ cup apple juice concentrate
$\frac{1}{2}$ tsp. cinnamon

Combine all ingredients and marinate for at least 4 hours before serving.

VARIATION:
Add 1 cup of grated raw apples just before serving. Or omit cinnamon and add 1 cup of finely chopped pineapple and 1 cup of thinly sliced celery.

Makes 12 servings. Each $\frac{1}{2}$-cup serving contains approximately 1 vegetable exchange, negligible fruit exchange, 35 calories.

3% fat
21 mg sodium
0 mg cholesterol

✗ CUCUMBER SALAD ✗

3 cucumbers, thinly sliced
1 red onion, thinly sliced

$\frac{1}{4}$ cup Peking Vinaigrette (see
p. 251)

Combine all ingredients.

Makes 4 servings of 1 cup each. Each serving contains approximately 1 vegetable exchange, 25 calories.

5% fat
6 mg sodium
0 mg cholesterol

✖ GREEN-BEAN SALAD ✖

5 cups green beans, broken into pieces
1 large red onion, thinly sliced

$\frac{1}{4}$ cup freshly squeezed lemon juice
$\frac{1}{4}$ Vinaigrette Dressing (see p. 252)

1. Steam the green beans until they are crisp and tender—about 5 minutes. Drain them thoroughly.
2. Combine the beans with the remaining ingredients and marinate for at least 4 hours before serving.

Makes 6 cups. Each 1-cup serving contains approximately 2 vegetable exchanges, 75 calories.

2% fat
13 mg sodium
0 mg cholesterol

✖ LEBANESE TABBOULI SALAD ✖

1 cup uncooked bulgur (cracked wheat)
Hot water to cover
$\frac{1}{4}$ cup lemon juice
$\frac{1}{2}$ tsp. low-sodium soy sauce
Dash cayenne pepper
1 clove garlic, minced

1 Tbsp. water
2 tomatoes, diced
1 cup minced parsley
1 cup chopped green onions
$\frac{1}{2}$ cup fresh finely chopped mint leaves
36 small romaine lettuce leaves

1. Soak the bulgur for 30 minutes in enough hot water to cover.
2. Meanwhile, combine the lemon juice, soy sauce, cayenne, garlic, and 1 Tbsp. of water. Mix well. Put dressing in a jar with a tight-fitting lid and shake vigorously for 30 seconds. Set aside.
3. Completely drain the bulgur. Add the tomatoes, parsley, green onions, and mint leaves to it. Add the dressing and toss thoroughly. Chill well.
4. On a chilled plate, surround each serving with 3 romaine leaves. (Traditionally this salad is eaten by scooping it up on the romaine leaves.)

Makes 12 servings. Each $\frac{1}{2}$-cup serving contains approximately $\frac{1}{2}$ complex-carbohydrate exchange, $\frac{1}{2}$ vegetable exchange, 50 calories.

4% fat
16 mg sodium
0 mg cholesterol

✶ MARINATED MUSHROOMS ✶

20 large mushrooms
2 Tbsp. fresh chopped parsley
2 Tbsp. sherry
$\frac{1}{2}$ cup Pritikin brand chicken broth

$\frac{1}{2}$ cup Pritikin brand Italian dressing
$\frac{1}{4}$ tsp. tamari
Garlic powder to taste

1. "Sauté" mushrooms and parsley in sherry in a sauté pan for a few minutes.
2. Remove from heat, transfer to a bowl, add the rest of the ingredients, and marinate for 1 hour.

Makes 4 servings. Each serving contains approximately 1 vegetable exchange, 40 calories.

7% fat
121 mg sodium
0 mg cholesterol

✶ MUSHROOM ANTIPASTO ✶

$1\frac{1}{4}$ cups tomato puree
$\frac{1}{2}$ cup water
2 Tbsp. red wine vinegar
1 tsp. toasted dehydrated onion flakes
1 clove garlic, minced
$\frac{1}{2}$ green pepper, seeded and diced

$\frac{1}{2}$ red pepper, seeded and diced
$\frac{1}{4}$ cup chopped fresh parsley
1 tsp. salad herbs or Italian herb blend
2 Tbsp. apple juice concentrate
$\frac{1}{4}$ tsp. freshly ground nutmeg
1 pound small fresh mushrooms, quartered

1. Combine tomato puree and water.
2. Then combine with all other ingredients except mushrooms and mix thoroughly. Pour over mushrooms and marinate overnight. Serve as hors d'oeuvres or antipasto.

Makes 4 servings. Each 1-cup serving contains approximately 3 vegetable exchanges, 75 calories.

6% fat
26 mg sodium
0 mg cholesterol

✖ PEKING VINAIGRETTE ✖

1 clove garlic
1 cup rice vinegar

Grating of fresh ginger
$\frac{1}{2}$ tsp. low-sodium soy sauce

Smash the garlic clove, but do not break it apart. Mix all the ingredients together and let them stand for 1 hour. Strain and serve over greens.

Makes 1 cup. Each 2-Tbsp. serving contains approximately 5 calories.

1% fat
85 mg sodium
0 mg cholesterol

✖ TUNA SALAD ✖

1 7-oz. can water-packed tuna, rinsed and drained
1 cup chopped celery
1 large green onion, chopped
$\frac{1}{2}$ cup chopped green bell pepper
$\frac{1}{2}$ cup chopped red bell pepper
2 cups bean sprouts

2 hard-cooked egg whites, chopped
1 large apple, cored and grated
$\frac{1}{2}$ cup Pritikin brand Italian dressing
2 Tbsp. Dijon mustard

1. Place tuna in a large bowl and flake with a fork. Add all remaining ingredients except the dressing and mustard and mix well.
2. Combine dressing and mustard, mixing well. Pour over tuna mixture and toss.

Makes 4 servings. Each serving contains approximately $\frac{1}{2}$ fruit exchange, 1 vegetable exchange, $1\frac{1}{2}$ oz. high protein, 160 calories.

VARIATION:
Omit Pritikin brand Italian dressing and Dijon mustard. Combine 4 Tbsp. water, 4 Tbsp. red wine vinegar, 2 tsp. unsalted Dijon mustard, and 1 tsp. Italian seasoning blend and use in Step 2 above.

5% fat
98 mg sodium
31 mg cholesterol

✖ VINAIGRETTE DRESSING ✖

1 cup dry white beans
Water
1 cup wine vinegar
2 garlic cloves, finely chopped

$\frac{1}{2}$ tsp. dry mustard
$\frac{1}{2}$ tsp. crushed basil
$\frac{1}{2}$ tsp. crushed rosemary

1. Cover beans with water and soak overnight.
2. Drain soaked beans and cover with fresh water in a pan. Bring to a boil.
3. Reduce the heat and simmer until tender, at least 1 hour. Cool to room temperature.
4. Combine cooked beans with remaining ingredients in a blender container. Blend until smooth.
5. Chill before using. Store in refrigerator in a jar with a tight-fitting lid.

Makes 3 cups. Each 2-Tbsp. serving contains approximately 20 calories.

2% fat
1 mg sodium
0 mg cholesterol

BEVERAGES

✖ CAFE OLÉ ✖

Prepare 8 oz. of hot grain beverage using steamed (or microwaved) nonfat milk instead of water. Sprinkle with cinnamon.

Makes 1 8-oz. serving. Each serving contains approximately 1 dairy exchange, negligible complex-carbohydrate exchange, 85 calories.

5% fat
93 mg sodium
4 mg cholesterol

✖ FRESH APPLE SODA ✖

$\frac{1}{4}$ cup apple juice concentrate
2 cups sparkling mineral water
   or no-salt-added seltzer

Ice
Apple slices (optional)
Cinnamon sticks (optional)

1. Combine apple juice concentrate and mineral water or seltzer and mix well.
2. Pour over ice and garnish with apple slices and cinnamon sticks if desired.

Makes 4 servings. Each serving contains approximately $\frac{1}{2}$ fruit exchange, 30 calories.

1% fat
4 mg sodium
0 mg cholesterol

✖ SPICED TEA ✖

2 cups boiling water
1 bag chamomile tea
1 bag red bush tea
1 Tbsp. apple juice concentrate
$\frac{1}{8}$ tsp. cardamom

2 cloves
$\frac{1}{8}$ tsp. ginger
2 1-inch pieces orange peel
2 small cinnamon sticks

1. Pour boiling water over the tea bags, apple juice concentrate, cardamom, cloves, and ginger. Let stand for 2 minutes.
2. Strain and pour into cups and serve with a piece of orange peel and a cinnamon stick.

Makes 2 servings. Each 1-cup serving contains negligible fruit exchange, approximately 25 calories.

6% fat
4 mg sodium
0 mg cholesterol

DESSERTS

✗ APPLE-DATE CAKE ✗

Nonstick cooking spray
1 cup whole-wheat flour
1 cup brown-rice flour
1 tsp. baking soda
1 tsp. baking powder
1 tsp. cinnamon
$\frac{1}{2}$ tsp. nutmeg
$\frac{1}{2}$ tsp. allspice
$\frac{1}{2}$ tsp. cloves

$\frac{1}{2}$ cup date sugar
2 cups applesauce, unsweetened
$\frac{1}{4}$ cup chopped dates
1 cup peeled, coarsely chopped apples
2 tsp. apple juice concentrate
1 tsp. vanilla
4 egg whites

1. Preheat oven to 350 degrees. Spray a nonstick tube pan with nonstick cooking spray.
2. In a large bowl, combine both flours with baking soda, baking powder, cinnamon, nutmeg, baking blend, and date sugar.
3. Add applesauce, dates, apples, apple juice concentrate, and vanilla. Mix well.
4. Beat egg whites in a separate bowl until they form soft peaks. Fold the beaten egg whites gently into the cake batter.
5. Pour the batter into the prepared tube pan and bake 50–60 minutes at 350 degrees, or until cake tester inserted in the center comes out clean.
6. Let cool a little. Loosen sides of cake gently with a spatula and unmold onto a cake platter. Allow to cool to room temperature before cutting.

Makes 12 servings. Each serving contains approximately $1\frac{1}{2}$ fruit exchanges, 1 complex-carbohydrate exchange, 165 calories.

2% fat
87 mg sodium
0 mg cholesterol

✄ BANANA "ICE CREAM" ✄

4 ripe bananas, peeled and sliced   Fresh mint sprigs (optional)
1 tsp. freshly grated orange peel
(optional)

1. Put sliced bananas in a plastic bag in the freezer.
2. When bananas are completely frozen, put into a food processor. Remove plunger to allow air to be incorporated. Blend until smooth.
3. Spoon frozen pureed bananas into 8 sherbet glasses and garnish with orange peel and mint if desired.

NOTE: Any type of acceptable extracts like vanilla, rum, or coconut can be added. Other fruits may be substituted for bananas but consistency is less creamy and more icy, or banana and another fruit such as pineapple or nectarine can be combined.

Makes 8 servings. Each serving contains approximately 1 fruit exchange, 55 calories.

VARIATION:
CAROB BANANA: Add 2 Tbsp. carob powder.

4% fat
1 mg sodium
0 mg cholesterol

✗ CHEESECAKE ✗

2 oz.	sprouted-grain bread	2 Tbsp.	vanilla extract
1	pound hoop cheese	1 tsp.	freshly grated lemon rind
$\frac{1}{2}$	cup nonfat milk	1 tsp.	fresh lemon juice
$\frac{1}{3}$	cup plus 3 Tbsp. apple juice concentrate		

1. Crumble bread and press evenly over the surface of a 9-inch pie plate.
2. Crumble the hoop cheese. Reserve $\frac{1}{4}$ cup for topping.
3. Put remaining hoop cheese, $\frac{1}{4}$ cup nonfat milk, $\frac{1}{3}$ cup apple juice concentrate, 1 Tbsp. vanilla, grated lemon rind, and lemon juice in a blender container. Blend until completely smooth.
4. Pour hoop-cheese mixture over the bread in the pie plate and spread evenly. Place in the center of a preheated 350-degree oven for 15 minutes.
5. While cheesecake is baking, combine the reserved $\frac{1}{4}$ cup hoop cheese, $\frac{1}{4}$ cup nonfat milk, 3 Tbsp. apple juice concentrate, and 1 Tbsp. vanilla extract in a blender container. Blend until completely smooth.
6. Remove cheesecake from oven and spread topping evenly over the surface. Place the cheesecake back into the oven and continue baking for another 10 minutes.
7. Cool to room temperature on a wire rack. Refrigerate until chilled before serving.

Makes 8 servings. Each serving contains approximately $\frac{1}{2}$ dairy exchange, negligible complex-carbohydrate exchange, 100 calories.

VARIATION:
BLUEBERRY CHEESECAKE: Add 1 cup of frozen unsweetened blueberries, unthawed, to the topping ingredients in Step 5 and mix thoroughly. This will add $\frac{1}{4}$ fruit exchange and 10 calories to each serving.

7% fat   2 mg cholesterol
46 mg sodium

✖ FLAN ✖

$\frac{1}{2}$ cup apple juice concentrate
$\frac{1}{2}$ tsp. cinnamon
3 Tbsp. cornstarch
$\frac{1}{4}$ cup water
$2\frac{1}{2}$ cups nonfat milk

$\frac{1}{2}$ cup plus 1 Tbsp. egg whites
1 tsp. vanilla
1 tsp. finely grated lemon rind
Fresh sliced fruit (optional)

1. Mix $\frac{1}{4}$ cup apple juice concentrate with the cinnamon. Heat until cinnamon is dissolved. Set aside.
2. Blend cornstarch with the water to dissolve. Put the remaining $\frac{1}{4}$ cup apple juice concentrate, milk, egg whites, vanilla, and lemon rind into a small saucepan. Add the cornstarch mixture and cook over medium heat, stirring constantly until thickened. Mixture should first come to a boil.
3. Coat six sherbet glasses with the set-aside apple juice/cinnamon syrup that has been equally divided.
4. Put thickened custard into coated sherbet glasses and refrigerate for several hours.
5. Garnish with fresh fruit slices if desired.

Makes 6 servings. Each serving contains approximately $\frac{1}{2}$ dairy exchange, 1 fruit exchange, 100 calories.

2% fat
99 mg sodium
40 mg cholesterol

✗ FROZEN BLUEBERRY CUSTARD ✗

1 envelope unflavored gelatin	$1\frac{1}{2}$ tsp. vanilla extract
2 Tbsp. cool water	2 tsp. lemon juice
$\frac{1}{4}$ cup boiling water	$\frac{1}{4}$ cup water
1 cup hoop cheese	$1\frac{1}{2}$ cups frozen unsweetened
3 Tbsp. powdered nonfat milk	blueberries, unthawed
2 Tbsp. apple juice concentrate	

1. Soften gelatin in the 2 Tbsp. of cool water and allow to stand for 5 minutes. Add the boiling water and stir until gelatin is completely dissolved. Cool for a few minutes.
2. Put hoop cheese, powdered milk, apple juice concentrate, vanilla extract, lemon juice, and gelatin mixture in a food processor. Blend until completely smooth.
3. Pour mixture into a bowl, cover, and refrigerate until jelled firmly.
4. Pour the $\frac{1}{4}$ cup water into blender container. Add jelled hoop cheese mixture and frozen blueberries to water in blender. It is important that water be placed in blender first so that it mixes more easily. Blend until smooth.

Makes 6 servings. Each $\frac{1}{2}$-cup serving contains approximately $\frac{1}{2}$ dairy exchange, $\frac{1}{2}$ fruit exchange, 90 calories.

VARIATION:
Any frozen fruit may be used in place of blueberries.

5% fat
31 mg sodium
2 mg cholesterol

✖ JEWEL-OF-FRUIT PIE ✖

$\frac{1}{2}$ cup plus 1 Tbsp. nugget
   cereal
2 bananas, ripe
$\frac{1}{3}$ cup apple juice concentrate
$\frac{1}{2}$ cup water
2 Tbsp. cornstarch
$1\frac{1}{2}$ cups black cherries, frozen
   and partially thawed

$1\frac{1}{2}$ cups strawberries, frozen and
   partially thawed
$1\frac{1}{2}$ cups blueberries, frozen and
   partially thawed
1 medium apple, grated

1. Sprinkle a layer of nugget cereal ($\frac{1}{2}$ cup) to evenly cover the bottom of a 10-inch French tart pan.
2. Slice the bananas lengthwise and place over the crust.
3. Combine the apple juice concentrate, water, and cornstarch in a saucepan. Cook until thickened.
4. Stir the thawed fruit and grated apple into the cornstarch mixture. Pour it over the bananas and spread it evenly. Sprinkle 1 Tbsp. of the nugget cereal on top for a strudel effect.
5. Bake in a 350-degree oven for 45 minutes. Serve at room temperature or refrigerate and serve the following day.

NOTE: Other unsweetened frozen fruit or fresh fruit may be substituted. A combination is best.

Makes 8 servings. Each serving contains approximately $1\frac{1}{2}$ fruit exchanges, $\frac{1}{2}$ complex-carbohydrate exchange, 130 calories.

3% fat   0 mg cholesterol
60 mg sodium

✖ PIÑA COLADA FROZEN YOGURT ✖

16 oz. plain nonfat yogurt
1 cup liquid nonfat milk
$\frac{3}{4}$ cup powdered nonfat milk
1 tsp. coconut extract

1 6-oz. can unsweetened
   pineapple juice concentrate
1 banana, very ripe
1 tsp. rum extract

1. Put all the ingredients in a blender or food processor and blend until smooth.
2. Place in an ice cream maker and follow manufacturer's instructions.

Makes 10 servings. Each serving contains approximately $\frac{1}{2}$ dairy exchange, $\frac{1}{2}$ fruit exchange, 90 calories.

2% fat   2 mg cholesterol
64 mg sodium

✄ STRAWBERRY-YOGURT CREME ✄

6 cups fresh strawberries, washed   Pinch cinnamon
   with stems removed   2 cups Yogurt Cheese (without
$\frac{1}{2}$ cup apple juice concentrate   herbs—see next recipe)
1 banana, mashed   Whoopee Topping (see p. 270)

1. Reserve 12 whole strawberries. Slice 3 cups of berries and marinate in $\frac{1}{4}$ cup of apple juice concentrate in the refrigerator for 2 hours.
2. Fold mashed banana and cinnamon into Yogurt Cheese. Fold in sliced strawberries marinated in the apple juice concentrate (include the juice).
3. Place the remaining strawberries (still reserving the 12) and the remaining $\frac{1}{4}$ cup apple juice concentrate into a blender and blend well to make a sauce.
4. To assemble, place some Strawberry-Yogurt Creme mixture into each of 12 tall parfait glasses. Follow with a layer of sauce, then more creme, continuing until the ingredients are used. Top with Whoopee Topping and more cinnamon. Garnish each glass with a whole berry.

Makes 12 servings. Each serving contains approximately $\frac{1}{2}$ dairy exchange, 1 fruit exchange, 105 calories.

4% fat
33 mg sodium
1 mg cholesterol

✖ YOGURT CHEESE ✖

1 quart homemade or
  commercial nonfat yogurt

1. Line a strainer with 3 thicknesses of cheesecloth. Drain the yogurt in the refrigerator overnight.
2. If desired, season the remaining curd with fresh dill or chives, mixing well.

Makes $1\frac{1}{2}$ cups. Each 2-Tbsp. serving contains approximately $\frac{1}{2}$ dairy exchange, 40 calories.

3% fat
29 mg sodium
1 mg cholesterol

✖ YOGURT PARFAIT ✖

6 oz. or $\frac{2}{3}$ cup plain nonfat
       yogurt
2   tsp. apple juice concentrate

1 tsp. vanilla
1 Tbsp. nugget cereal
$\frac{1}{2}$ cup fresh fruit or berries

1. Combine yogurt with apple juice concentrate and vanilla.
2. Place half of the nugget cereal in the bottom of a parfait glass or sundae dish.
3. Spoon half of the yogurt into the dish.
4. Add the fresh fruit or berries (reserving a few) and top with the remaining yogurt. Sprinkle the remaining nugget cereal and reserved fruit on top to garnish.

Makes 1 serving. Each serving contains approximately 1 dairy exchange, 1 fruit exchange, negligible complex-carbohydrate exchange, 185 calories.

3% fat
172 mg sodium
3 mg cholesterol

SAUCES, DIPS, TOPPINGS, AND CONDIMENTS

✖ CHUTNEY ✖

1 pound tart green apples, peeled, cored, and diced	1 tsp. onion powder
1 medium onion, peeled and diced	$\frac{1}{2}$ tsp. ground mustard
$\frac{1}{2}$ cup finely chopped dried figs	$\frac{1}{2}$ tsp. chili powder
$\frac{1}{4}$ cup raisins	$1\frac{1}{2}$ tsp. ground ginger
1 cup cider vinegar	$\frac{1}{4}$ tsp. cayenne pepper
1 6-oz. can apple juice concentrate, undiluted	1 Tbsp. pickling spices, tied in a cheesecloth bag

1. Combine all ingredients in a large saucepan. Bring to a boil, reduce heat, and simmer slowly, uncovered, for 2 hours.
2. Cool to room temperature. Remove and discard spice bag. Store covered in the refrigerator.

Makes 2 cups. Each 2-Tbsp. serving contains approximately $1\frac{1}{2}$ fruit exchanges, 90 calories.

4% fat
6 mg sodium
0 mg cholesterol

✖ DILL SAUCE ✖

1 cup nonfat yogurt	1 Tbsp. crushed dill weed
1 tsp. crushed tarragon	$\frac{1}{2}$ tsp. low-sodium soy sauce

Combine all ingredients in a bowl and mix thoroughly. Store, covered, in refrigerator. (For best results, prepare a day in advance.)

Makes 4 servings. Each $\frac{1}{4}$-cup serving contains approximately $\frac{1}{3}$ dairy exchange, 45 calories.

4% fat
65 mg sodium
1 mg cholesterol

✗ FRUIT SYRUP ✗

1 16-oz. package unsweetened
frozen fruit, thawed

1–2 Tbsp. apple juice concentrate

Blend thawed fruit and apple juice concentrate together in a food processor until pureed.

Makes 4 servings. Each $\frac{1}{2}$-cup serving contains approximately 1 fruit exchange, 60 calories.

1% fat
4 mg sodium
0 mg cholesterol

✗ HOT CINNAMON APPLESAUCE ✗

¼ cup unsweetened applesauce
cinnamon to taste

Heat $\frac{1}{4}$ cup unsweetened applesauce over medium flame. Add cinnamon to taste. Makes excellent topping for whole-wheat pancakes or waffles, toasted bagel, etc.

Makes 1 serving. Each serving contains approximately $\frac{1}{2}$ fruit exchange, 30 calories.

1% fat
2 mg sodium
0 mg cholesterol

✗ MARINARA SAUCE ✗

2 Tbsp. defatted chicken stock
1 small onion, finely chopped
2 cloves garlic, finely chopped
1 small carrot, grated
3 pounds fresh tomatoes, peeled
  and seeded, or 1 28-oz. can
  Italian plum tomatoes

4 Tbsp. chopped fresh basil, or 2
  Tbsp. crushed dried basil
2 Tbsp. chopped Italian parsley
3 Tbsp. tomato paste
2 Tbsp. grated sapsago cheese,
  toasted
2 Tbsp. Italian seasoning

1. Heat the chicken stock in a large saucepan. Add the onion, garlic, and carrot and "sauté" for 5 minutes.
2. Coarsely chop the tomatoes and add them to the saucepan. Add the remaining ingredients and simmer slowly for 1 hour.
3. Puree in a blender or use a food processor for a more textured sauce.

Makes 6 servings. Each 1-cup serving contains approximately 3 vegetable exchanges, 75 calories.

8% fat
28 mg sodium
0 mg cholesterol

✗ MOCK SOUR CREAM ✗

2 cups low-fat (1%) cottage
  cheese
$\frac{1}{4}$ cup nonfat yogurt or nonfat
  buttermilk

$\frac{1}{2}$ tsp. onion powder (optional)
$\frac{1}{2}$ tsp. garlic powder (optional)
$\frac{1}{2}$ tsp. lemon juice (optional)
Fresh or dried chives (optional)

1. Combine the cottage cheese and yogurt or buttermilk in a food processor.
2. Add spices if desired. With a spoon or spatula, *fold in* the chives if desired (do not use the food processor or the mixture will turn green).

VARIATION:
Mock Sour Cream is a versatile food. Vary the spices added according to its use. For baked potatoes, definitely add chives. As a topping for soup, leave it rich and simple.

Makes about 2 cups. Each 2-Tbsp. serving contains negligible dairy exchange, approximately 20 calories.

10% fat
52 mg sodium
1 mg cholesterol

TORTILLA CHIPS

12 corn tortillas
Onion powder, garlic powder, or
other seasoning mixture

1. Cut each tortilla into 6 or 8 pie-shaped wedges (3 or 4 tortillas can be cut at the same time).
2. Preheat oven to 400 degrees. Spread the tortilla chips on a baking sheet or cookie tray in a single layer. Don't overlap. Lightly mist with water so seasonings will adhere. Sprinkle on desired seasonings. Bake for 7 to 8 minutes until crisp. Remove from oven and let cool. Store in an airtight container.

NOTE: To freshen stale chips, place on a baking sheet and reheat in a 350-degree oven for about 5 minutes or until crisp.

Makes 72–96 chips; 9–12 chips ($1\frac{1}{2}$ tortillas) contain approximately 1 complex-carbohydrate exchange, 100 calories.

7% fat
79 mg sodium
0 mg cholesterol

✖ WHOOPEE TOPPING ✖

1 cup liquid nonfat milk, chilled in freezer until ice crystals just start to form

1 tsp. vanilla extract
2 Tbsp. apple juice concentrate

1. Chill a mixing bowl and rotary beaters for an electric mixer in the freezer.
2. Combine all the ingredients in the chilled bowl and whip with the chilled beaters until the mixture is the desired consistency. Serve immediately.

Makes approximately 5 cups. Each 2-Tbsp. serving contains negligible dairy exchange, approximately 10 calories.

VARIATIONS:
Combine all ingredients in a food processor. Remove the plunger. Whip until thick.

4% fat
11 mg sodium
0 mg cholesterol

CHAPTER 14

Let's Eat Out!

What about dining out?

By now, you've got a very clear idea of what the Lifetime Eating Plan is all about, and, in fact, you can probably figure out a great deal of what "eating out" according to the Pritikin program guidelines entails. Our main purpose here is to remind you how easy it can be to enjoy delicious meals outside your own home, and to give you a few tips to help you along—reminders, really, that you've got more restaurant options (whether you're at the corner coffee shop or a trendy bistro) than you may have thought you did! Sure, the old temptations will be there—fried food, buttery pastries, fatty meats—but there are so many healthy and delicious alternatives there, too, that you'll be able to navigate past the "bad stuff" without regret. We promise!

We'll give you a quick rundown of general tips that apply wherever you eat out, then a meal-by-meal breakdown (from breakfast to dinner, including buffets) of what to look out for, and then some handy "Poor," "Better," and "Best" choices you're apt to find on your favorite ethnic food menu (yes, you *can* eat out at Chinese, Mexican, Italian, and French restaurants!). You're already getting to be a pro at the Pritikin plan—this will just help you succeed in a restaurant as well as you're already succeeding in your own kitchen!

271

FIVE TIPS FOR EATING OUT

A lot of this is just common sense, but all of it is geared to help you to eat out healthfully and enjoyably wherever you go.

1. Plan Ahead.

The way to choose a restaurant is on the basis of how easy it will be to eat there the way *you* want to eat. Keep a mental (or even written) list of restaurants you've gone to (or which you'd like to try) whose menus include foods you know are good for you: This might include your local steak house (almost all offer fish or chicken and a baked potato without butter or sour cream), or restaurants whose fish or meat portions aren't so huge that you'd be tempted to eat more than the optimal $3\frac{1}{2}$ ounces. (Remember, of course, that you can always halve your portion discreetly and take the rest home for tomorrow night's dinner.) Just keep your favorite healthy restaurants in mind so when your friends suggest going out to dinner you'll be ready with a few good ideas about where to go.

Another way to plan ahead is to be prepared for a spontaneous stop at a diner or restaurant by keeping a few packets of oil-free salad dressing, seasonings, or herb tea bags on hand in your briefcase, glove compartment, or purse.

2. Be Adventurous—Choose New Foods from the Menu!

You don't have to resign yourself to the "same old" boiled or baked potatoes, broiled fish and chicken, and steamed vegetables. Look for unusual dishes—perhaps vegetables and fruits you've never tried before, but that you know fall within healthy guidelines. Try new kinds of squash, order an artichoke, or try an "exotic" fish like mahimahi or poached chicken with an unusual fruit sauce. Open your mind to new taste sensations! We do tend to limit ourselves (and then feel "deprived") unnecessarily, forgetting that there really are a lot of things to choose from. Just look at the menu creatively, and try something new!

3. Be Clear about Your Needs.

A friendly server is one of the greatest assets you can have in a restaurant, and luckily, there are a lot of friendly servers. Enlist him or her as your ally, explaining that you're after something "wonderful" that doesn't include butter, oil, or other fats, or added salt. (Remember that it's not enough to say "Hold the butter": You might end up with *cheese* sauce dumped on your vegetables anyway!) A good tactic is to ask your server's opinion—what would he or she choose from the menu if he or she were on a low-fat, low-sodium diet? (Maybe your server is!) Once you've won your server over, he or she will most likely get the chef to oblige you by poaching the fillet of sole instead of broiling it in butter—or by preparing other dishes more healthfully, even if they aren't listed that way on the menu.

In fact, here are a few things you can usually count on getting at a restaurant if you ask—alternatives that your server will normally be happy to bring you:

- Salad dressing or sauce on the side (in case it's oily), or fresh lemon, lime, or vinegar in place of an oily dressing.
- If it's available, plain nonfat yogurt with chopped chives or some salsa instead of sour cream or butter for baked potatoes.
- Meat, fish, or poultry that's baked, braised, steamed, poached in wine or stock, or broiled or grilled without butter or oil, instead of sautéed or deep-fried.
- A smaller portion of meat, fish, or poultry and a larger serving of vegetables and starchy foods such as potatoes, steamed rice, or pasta.
- Dishes prepared without added salt or MSG.
- Sliced tomatoes or a baked or boiled potato instead of french fries or chips.
- A sandwich prepared with mustard or tomato slices instead of mayonnaise, butter, or margarine.
- Fresh fruit or sorbet instead of cake or pie for dessert.

4. Work from the Entire Menu.

You may feel needlessly restricted if you don't see anything suitable in the entrees—so why not select from the first courses and appetizers? Perhaps a soup and salad plus an appetizer? Can you order the vegetable of the day? There are usually a lot of ways to create a delicious, satisfying meal by picking and choosing from smaller first courses—in the spirit of what the Spanish call *tapas*—and sometimes you will end up with a much more interesting meal than if you had simply ordered an entree.

5.　If You Have to Compromise, Compromise with Care.
A common psychological trick your mind can play on you runs as follows: You look at the menu—it seems everything has butter cooked right into it! The meats are stuffed with pâté . . . bacon garnishes the vegetables . . . the potatoes come with cheese. There doesn't seem to be anything you can eat! So (the trick goes) what can you do? You have to eat, don't you? You might as well give up and have that 16-ounce steak with foie gras, the fried onions, the chocolate mousse . . .

Wait! Remember the "Stop," "Caution," and "Go" food categories, and take some time to weigh your options: You'll almost always find that there are healthier choices on the menu if you look for them. If everything is cooked with oil, choose something with a "Caution" oil like olive oil. And remember the substitution tips we just gave you—ask for sauces to be put on the side. Eating out may sometimes mean you'll have to dip into the "Caution" category, but it doesn't mean you have to give up and plunge into "Stop"!

RESTAURANT BASICS—FOR ANY MEAL OF THE DAY

Here are some pointers and reminders about making breakfast, lunch, and dinner satisfying *and* healthy when you eat out—plus a word about buffets, which you can easily turn into a healthy feast.

Breakfast
This is one of the easiest meals to adapt to Pritikin plan guidelines. Cold cereals like shredded-wheat biscuits, puffed wheat or rice, and nugget cereal, or hot cereal like oatmeal (farina and corn grits are second choices since they're "refined" grains), are all fine, with skim milk: Already you've got the central part of a satisfying morning meal. (If skim milk isn't available, you might want to try fruit juice on your cereal.) Add fresh fruit as a topping for your cereal (or order it to have on the side); remember, it's better than fruit juice because it provides more fiber and fewer calories. Then have a slice or two of whole-wheat toast with a little jam, and hot herb tea—again, be prepared with your own herb tea bag in case they don't have it, or ask for hot water with fresh lemon, which makes a re-

freshing breakfast drink. You're all set! If you want eggs, order them poached or hard-boiled so you can set aside the yolks and enjoy the whites. The pancakes and waffles served in restaurants are usually made with whole eggs, so it's best to pass them up.

Or be inventive! If the restaurant isn't packed and frantic, and if it seems like a friendly place, ask for an egg-white omelet. Or perhaps they'd make up a terrific breakfast or brunch sandwich with the chopped whites of hard-boiled eggs and sliced tomatoes, lettuce, peppers, and mustard on a no-egg bagel: It's delicious! Another custom-tailored breakfast might be huevos rancheros, a Mexican dish popular in the West but popping up in various forms all over the country: Ask for a steamed (not fried) tortilla, topped with boiled (rather than refried) beans with some salsa or picante sauce, or chopped egg white. You might even be able to order baked or boiled potatoes to have with scrambled egg whites and chives or mushrooms—the worst they can say is no, and you may be introducing them to new dishes they'll end up offering regularly! Don't be shy; it's worth a try.

Lunch

Follow the same guidelines at lunch that you would in your own kitchen: You'll find, whatever the restaurant, that it's not hard at all! Your special ally is always a salad bar; use it to supplement some chicken and a potato so you can have a big, filling meal, or turn to it for your *whole* lunch. We're not saying that salad greens alone make a meal, but garbanzo beans (chick-peas), kidney beans, and pasta or rice with chopped egg whites, onions, beets, sprouts, salsa, and no-salt seasonings like vinegar, garlic powder, and oregano *do!* Remember the satisfying baked potato, and how many toppings you can use to zip it up—from nonfat yogurt and chives to chili beans, tomatoes, or ratatouille.

Have a sandwich if you want: Choose a whole-grain bread or whole-wheat pita, ask for a little mustard and shredded vegetables to go with your chicken or turkey breast, and you've got a great lunch. An overstuffed veggie sandwich in a pita pocket is a great idea, too—with a few splashes of vinegar to perk it up. As for soups, stick to the clear broth-based soups (not the creamy kinds) like chicken with rice, or minestrone. These soups, as well as most commercial brands of bean and lentil soups, *do* tend to be high in sodium, however, so regard them as "Caution" choices.

Dinner
Follow the guidelines for lunch and you've pretty much got dinner! Remember to request that your chicken or fish be poached or broiled without butter, instead of fried, and remember the wonderful (if misleadingly named) restaurant amenity called the "doggy bag," which will enable you to take home the other half of an overly large portion of meat or fish. Or you might be able to share an entree with one of your companions, and order an extra potato or serving of rice or pasta. As for dessert (this obviously applies to lunch, too), check to see if they've got a baked apple or pear without butter or whipped cream; otherwise fresh fruit remains your best choice.

Buffets
These popular "smorgasbord" meals deserve special mention because they so frequently offer a rich array of healthy foods, as well as tempt you with many of the unhealthy foods you're trying to avoid. Follow all the guidelines we've already set out, but do look for some special treats in the buffet lineup so you won't feel deprived when you pass up the Swedish meatballs! You might find rice dishes without fat, scallops with lemon, oysters on the half-shell, turkey or chicken breast without the skin, pastas with tomato-based sauces, or pasta primavera (with fresh vegetables, but no cream). You're quite apt to find bagels and fresh fruit at a breakfast or brunch buffet, or perhaps you could ask for an egg-white omelet if eggs are being made to order. It's always a good idea to check on how things have been prepared; then, of course, select those foods which are in their natural state (or as close to it as possible). This is particularly applicable to salads, which usually abound at buffets (sometimes with unusual greens you may never have tried before)—so indulge yourself freely as long as they aren't bathed in fatty dressings.

EASY EATING À LA CARTE

Now let's put all this together. Say you're away from home on a business trip for four days. No shopping, no dishes! What might a typical four-day collection of basic restaurant meals be? Here are some suggestions:

DAY 1

Breakfast	*Lunch*	*Dinner*
Wheat-biscuit cereal with nonfat milk and blueberries (or other fresh fruit); fresh-squeezed orange or grapefruit juice; 2 slices whole-wheat toast with fruit spread	Roast turkey sandwich ($3\frac{1}{2}$ oz. white meat) on whole-grain bread with mustard, lettuce, tomato, sprouts; vegetable barley soup; nonfat milk	"Buddha's Delight" (steamed vegetables), steamed rice, Chinese noodle soup; fresh mandarin orange and pineapple slices

DAY 2

Breakfast	*Lunch*	*Dinner*
Hard-boiled egg-white sandwich on water bagel with lettuce and tomato; fresh fruit salad; nonfat milk	Cheeseless pizza with peppers, onions, tomatoes, mushrooms; green salad with red wine vinegar; fresh fruit	$3\frac{1}{2}$ oz. white salmon with dill and lemon; steamed artichoke (or other vegetable) with vinaigrette; salad of endive and yellow pepper; large baked potato with nonfat yogurt and chives; French bread; baked apple

DAY 3

Breakfast	*Lunch*	*Dinner*
Hot oatmeal with cinnamon and nonfat milk;	Salad bar: assorted raw veggies, kidney beans, garbanzos,	Salad with balsamic vinegar; chicken breast sautéed in

DAY 3 (continued)

Breakfast	*Lunch*	*Dinner*
honeydew melon; English muffin with fruit spread	corn, peas, hard-cooked egg white; baked potato with salsa; tomato rice soup with a roll; fresh pineapple	wine with mushrooms; steamed broccoli with lemon; peas and pearl onions; steamed red potatoes; French bread; raspberry sorbet

DAY 4

Breakfast	*Lunch*	*Dinner*
Egg-white omelet with onions and peppers; whole-wheat toast with fruit preserves or applesauce; nonfat milk; broiled grapefruit	Bowl of minestrone soup; pasta with basil and marinara sauce; green salad with garbanzo beans; nectarine	Soft chicken tacos (no cheese) with lettuce, chopped tomatoes, and onions; boiled beans; gazpacho; grapes and orange slices

ETHNIC RESTAURANTS

Does following healthy food guidelines mean you have to stop eating at your favorite Italian, Chinese, French, and Mexican restaurants? Absolutely not! As you'll see from the following tips and menu suggestions, you can enjoy a variety of dishes from all these cuisines, without fear of "slipping." Read on and see how easy it is to ensure that your "international" dining is as delicious *and* as healthy as possible.

Italian

Italian restaurants offer abundant opportunities to eat healthfully and well. Pasta, salad, and bread make a delightful dinner—high in complex carbohydrates, yet low in fat and cholesterol. Try to stick to spaghetti or linguine; very fine pastas (like cappellini, or "angel hair") and wide pastas (from fettucine to lasagna) tend to be made with egg. The best way to be sure is to ask.

As for sauces, you just might want to ask your server which sauce has the least oil; chances are, if any oil is used at all it will be olive oil—the least "dangerous" kind—but it's best to see if you can find a sauce that's oil-free, anyway. The better sauces tend to be marinara, Neapolitan tomato, or anything with a seafood/tomato base. Alfredo sauces, or any others with a cream or butter base, are obviously not recommended. One delightful possibility is pasta primavera—pasta tossed with fresh tomatoes (not fresh cream!) and vegetables.

Entrees of chicken, fish, or shellfish in a tomato-based sauce made without oil or fat are fine selections. They will probably be prepared with one or more of the wonderful Italian herbs and spices (like basil, oregano, fennel seed, or garlic), but ask that no salt be used. Or see if they'll make you a cheeseless pizza without olive oil and with peppers, onions, and mushrooms (or something a little more adventurous, like broccoli or artichoke hearts) in place of the mozzarella. (In Italy, pizza without cheese is common.) Enjoy your salad with lemon juice or balsamic vinegar, or try a little marinara sauce on your greens. It makes a wonderful salad dressing! Fresh fruit, as always, is a good dessert, and the perfect cap to an Italian meal.

Here are some sample menu choices, rated for desirability:

Poor:	breaded veal parmigiano
Better:	chicken cacciatore
Best:	eggless pasta with fresh vegetables and marinara sauce

Chinese

One of the happy basics of Chinese cooking is that most dishes are prepared separately, which means it's usually possible to have meals cooked to order. Ask that oil be replaced with water, juice, wine, or chicken broth in the wok for stir-frying, and that sugars, soy sauce, and MSG be omitted (long a staple in Chinese kitchens, MSG has become optional in more and more restaurants). The Chinese have exactly the right idea about using meat, fish, or poultry—small amounts to accent a dish rich in vegetables, rather than an enormous portion monopolizing your plate.

While steamed rice is a refined grain (ask if they've got brown rice, which many Chinese restaurants now do), it's a much better choice than fried rice, with its heavy soy-sauce and relatively high oil content. Order plain steamed vegetables with rice, vegetarian chop suey, or a popular vegetarian specialty called "Buddha's Delight." Other possibilities might be chicken chop suey, chow mein, lo mein (a soft noodle dish that is sometimes a bit greasy, so ask that it be prepared without oil), moo goo gai pan, or scallops or other seafood selections. Chinese teas *are* caffeinated—and are sometimes very strong—so this is a good time to have a few herbal tea bags on hand.

Typical Chinese restaurant choices, rated, would include:

Poor: egg foo yung

Better: beef chow fun with soft noodles (less than optimal if it contains oil and soy sauce)

Best: "Stir-fried" vegetables prepared in wine with ginger and garlic, and steamed rice (or "Buddha's Delight" with steamed rice)

Mexican

Mexican restaurants make use of foods that are potentially perfect on the Pritikin plan—corn tortillas, beans, salsa, and various fresh vegetables (especially chilies, other peppers, and tomatoes), along with white chicken meat and fish. The problem is making sure they're not deep-fried in fat. Corn tortillas are preferable since the ones made with wheat flour usually contain lard or some other kind of cholesterol-raising fat. Ask for steamed tortillas instead of the usual deep-fried chips that Mexican restaurants have on the table for nibbling. Call the restaurant in advance to see if they'll honor your request for a fat-free bean or rice dish (refried beans are prepared with lard, so see if you can get your beans boiled instead).

Good entree choices include enchiladas—corn tortillas filled with seasoned chicken and a mild tomato sauce. To replace the cheese, sour cream, and guacamole toppings, ask for shredded lettuce, tomatoes, and other assorted fresh vegetables, along with onion slices and extra salsa (sometimes you can order a side dish of vegetables and add them yourself). Other good dishes: gazpacho, ceviche, chicken or bean tostadas, or taco salad (without the cheese, guacamole, sour cream, fried pastry shell, or taco chips). Fancier menu choices might be red snapper or a fleshy white fish served with a tomato sauce "à la Veracruzana."

Typical Mexican restaurant choices, rated:

Poor: chilis rellenos
Better: beef enchilada
Best: soft chicken tacos in steamed corn tortillas (without cheese), fresh salsa

Japanese

Like Chinese food, Japanese cuisine has a wonderful way of combining meat, vegetables, and starch (rice or noodles) in optimal proportions. The problem with Japanese food is all the soy sauce, and thus the extremely high sodium content of many of its dishes. In small amounts, and especially if it's sodium-reduced, soy sauce is a "Caution" condiment, so try to choose dishes that don't depend too heavily on it (dipping sauces are usually 90 percent soy sauce, so be wary of them). Do ask, as you will in Chinese restaurants, that oil, salt, sugar, and MSG be omitted from your meal. Small amounts (half a teaspoon) of soy sauce or preferably garlic are the seasonings that can replace them.

Japanese restaurants usually feature marvelous seafood entrees, like halibut simmered in broth, as well as sushi and sashimi, which have become so popular in recent years. (Do be aware, however, that there is a danger of parasites in raw fish. Experts recommend avoiding bargain or buffet sushi, and staying with the highest-quality restaurants to ensure safety.) Traditional one-pot dishes are also wonderful, such as mizutake, which typically contains cabbage, carrots, watercress, mushrooms, tofu, and small pieces of chicken, or chicken sukiyaki (ask to have the skin removed ahead of time or remove it yourself); you can also order vegetarian versions with tofu only. Some Japanese restaurants or sushi bars may feature grilled vegetables like yams or eggplant, with their skins (and nutrients) intact. If the vegetables are grilled with fat, you can simply remove the skins and eat the fiber-rich vegetable inside. Salads are usually tossed with a dressing; ask for yours with just vinegar or lemon wedges.

Typical Japanese menu choices, rated:

Poor: shrimp tempura
Better: teriyaki chicken
Best: vegetable sukiyaki (with light soy sauce)

French

The words to look for on a French menu are *poached, steamed, baked, broiled,* or *roasted.* Since these are popular French cooking techniques, you can already see the wide range of choices open to you! As always, avoid butter and ask that oil be left out or kept to a minimum. Start your French meal with some consommé or a tomato-based vegetable or lentil soup. Ask for lemon juice or for wine, rasperry, or balsamic vinegar to dress salads as well as fresh raw or steamed vegetables.

For entrees, consider poached or broiled salmon, roasted chicken (remember to remove the skin), or a tuna niçoise salad (without oil or egg yolk). There are usually plenty of fresh vegetables to choose from: asparagus, artichokes, baby peas, and more. Delicious vegetable dishes might include mushrooms simmered in wine, ratatouille, tomato and onion salad with fresh herbs, and baked zucchini, eggplant, or tomatoes. Avoid quiche and crepes, since they contain all the high-cholesterol and high-fat ingredients you want to avoid—whole eggs, cream, bacon, and butter. French bread, like Italian, is usually baked without eggs or oil, and, although it's made from "refined" grain, it's an acceptable accompaniment to a French meal. Fresh fruit, as always, makes a great dessert—but see if they offer a fruit sorbet as a change and a treat.

Typical French restaurant choices, rated:

Poor: quiche lorraine
Better: roast lamb with rosemary
Best: poached salmon with mushrooms "sautéed" in wine

FAST-FOOD RESTAURANTS

What about all those quick burger and chicken chain restaurants that continue to tempt you? Is it possible to maneuver your way successfully through the typical fast-food menu?

It's a testament to the growing food consciousness of the American public that fast-food restaurants are waking up and offering some healthy alternatives to the greasy fare with which they're usually associated: Now, at least, there are some relatively healthy choices beyond quarter-pound cheeseburgers, fries, and shakes. Breakfast is perhaps the worst, since fast-food breakfast sandwiches are usually fat and cholesterol horrors: fatty meat *and* cheese *and* egg! The best alternative might be an English muffin—have it without butter but with a little jam—and some fruit juice.

Lunch and dinner offer more variety. Look for the growing number of serve-yourself salad bars and follow the guidelines we've already given you for making a good meal from a salad bar. Some fast-food restaurants now offer roasted or broiled chicken sandwiches, which are far better choices than deep-fried chicken nuggets: Add tomatoes, lettuce, and mustard for flavor—and a little extra nutrition. Baked potatoes, corn on the cob, chicken, or garden salad with your own packet of dressing brought from home—options higher in nutrition now abound in many fast-food places, so don't give in to fries!

SIT BACK AND RELAX

To sum up, here are thirteen tips for smart—and pleasurable—restaurant dining:

1. Have a plan.
2. Be ready with suggestions for appropriate restaurants.
3. Call ahead to request specially prepared foods if necessary.
4. Ask your server questions about the foods and how they're prepared.
5. Be assertive—but polite—about your order (get your server on your side!).
6. Politely return food if not prepared as you requested. Be ready to explain your order more clearly.
7. Enjoy the sociability of dining as well as the food—concentrate on the good company!
8. If portions are large, divide them before you begin to eat. Split a meat entree with your dining companions.
9. Request a "doggy bag" at the end of your meal to take home excess-portions.

10. Take "extras" with you in your purse or briefcase—salad-dressing packets, herb tea bags, seasonings, or even a small jar of fruit spread.
11. Accept the fact that you may have to dip into "Caution" foods when you eat out—not every dining experience will be perfect!
12. Show your gratitude when you receive special service.
13. Always maintain a sense of humor and a positive attitude. If the service or the food is lacking, don't let it become a source of stress or anger for you. Look forward to your *next* meal instead!

Fat City

For those times when you're not following the Lifetime Eating Plan, it's helpful to have a gauge to determine the impact of the higher-fat foods you may be eating. One good way to do this is to look at the grams of fat in the foods you select.

Here's how it would work: On a 1,500-calorie-per-day diet with 10 percent fat calories, 150 calories would come from fat (that would equal about $16\frac{1}{2}$ grams of fat, since there are 9 calories in a gram of fat).

Imagine you're doing well with your eating choices, but then decide to have a Danish pastry, which contains about 18 grams of fat. You just ate more than a whole day's fat allowance—and bumped the amount of fat in your diet right up to about 21 percent.

Here are some examples of common foods that quickly move you into "Fat City."

Source: Jean A. T. Pennington, *Bowes & Church's Food Values of Portions Commonly Used,* 15th ed. Philadelphia: Lippincott, 1989.

As you become more and more at ease with the Pritikin Lifetime Eating Plan, you'll find you can take it anywhere—not just to a restaurant downtown, but on the road, in the air, or overseas. Whether it's a week's vacation at the shore, an unanticipated business hop to another city, or a full-fledged European vacation, you can take your healthy eating plan with you. Holiday parties and dinners, traditionally replete with high-fat foods, are also navigable. If you need to be convinced, read the next chapter!

	Calories	Grams of Fat	% of Fat Calories	Approx. Cholesterol (mg)	Sodium (mg)
Large hamburger, reg. fries, mcd. vanilla shake	1,188	64	49	140	1,207
Double hamburger with cheese and mayonnaise-based sauce, reg. fries, med. chocolate shake	1,173	56	43	122	1,388
Fried chicken dinner (2 pcs. center-breast chicken, mashed potatoes with gravy, coleslaw, roll)	759	37	44	195	1,672
Double cheeseburger, reg. fries, med. soft-serve dessert	1,450	69	43	245	1,151
Taco	191	11	52	21	406
Fish sandwich	435	26	54	45	799

CHAPTER 15

Rising to ALL Occasions: Travel, Holidays, and Other Special Events

If you travel at all in the United States, you're aware of the good news that there's been what amounts to a revolution in nutritious food choices in markets, restaurants, and health-food stores almost everywhere you go. No longer are low-sodium and low-fat or nonfat foods limited to out-of-the-way specialty shops: As you've seen in previous chapters, supermarkets stock cereals, sauces, vegetables, pastas, and condiments that closely follow Pritikin plan guidelines (and don't forget that there's a line of Pritikin brand food products), and restaurants have never been more receptive to requests for healthy food. What all this means is that any trepidations you may have about eating healthfully wherever you go—on long or short trips—are really unnecessary: You can apply all the principles you've learned no matter where you are.

What this chapter will do is cover a few of the special-occasion challenges that might crop up when you travel by air or by car, not only in this country, but overseas as well. And what about holiday parties and meals—those you go to and those you host yourself? Won't they present special difficulties? Let's broaden our horizons a bit and show you that there's really *no* event, trip, party, or celebration that can't be made healthy.

THE PRITIKIN PLAN AT 30,000 FEET

You probably already know that you can request special meals when you fly the major airlines, but you may not know what a range of choices are available, or that some airlines offer things others do not. We won't give you an airline-by-airline breakdown here, because food offerings change too quickly; luckily, they've been changing in healthier directions, with more low-fat and low-cholesterol choices starting to abound. What we can report is that meal options usually include fruit plates and diabetic, seafood, low-fat, low-cholesterol, or strictly vegetarian dishes.

When you make your plane reservations, be sure to ask about specific foods on the menus since definitions of low-fat and low-cholesterol may vary from one airline to another. If the airline representative has the time, you might be able to outline an ideal meal: A salad with no-oil dressing (or lemon slices), a plain baked potato, steamed vegetables, nonfat milk, whole-wheat bread or rolls, and baked fish or broiled chicken. Then simply ask the agent to select the meal type that best corresponds to your request. Don't be shy (but do be flexible).

One other very important point is to call as far in advance as you can to place your order: Most airlines require a minimum of twenty-four hours' notice, but some may require more time than that—so to be safe, put in your request early, and call again to confirm it. When you board, identify yourself to the flight attendant as having ordered a special meal.

You also have the option of taking food on board *with* you—not a bad idea, especially if the flight isn't a long one, or you can't get what you want from the airline's menu. And don't get on board hungry! Refer to the following list of take-on foods before you fly—and when you'll be traveling by car, bus, or train, too!

Bread/Crackers
Pita bread
Pritikin brand rice cakes
Crackers (like matzo, rye crackers,
  brown-rice snaps)

Dairy
Dry nonfat milk packets

Fruit
Fresh fruit
Unsweetened fruit spread
Dried fruits without sulfites
Apple butter

Vegetables
Fresh vegetables cut up and stored
in plastic bags

High-Protein Animal
3-oz. can of water-packed tuna or
salmon

Beverages
Low-salt tomato or vegetable juice
Mineral water
Herb tea bags
Grain-beverage packets

Condiments
Low-sodium mustard
Hot pepper sauce
Pritikin brand individual portion
creamy Italian dressing
Salt-free seasoning blends

ON THE ROAD

The above list of carry-on snacks and foods is also perfect for traveling by car. However, because you may be spending a lot of time in your car if you're going on a long trip, and because you certainly have more room and autonomy in a car than you do on a plane, you've got a lot more options on the ground than you do in the air!

Think of your car as more than a means of transportation—think of it as your traveling "restaurant" and storage compartment: It gives you room to store healthy snacks (such as the ones listed above) that you can pack before you take off and replenish as you go along. A great way to appreciate the country you're driving through is to stop off at a roadside stand for some local fresh produce. Instead of eating at the usual fast-food or steam-table restaurants you'll find at highway rest stops, be adventurous: Drive off the main highway every so often and keep your eye open for interesting "natural-food" restaurants, cafés, and food stands. Or stop off at a market and pick up some good-food snacks. (Remember that the Pritikin Lifetime Eating Plan encourages you to eat regularly throughout the day.)

Here are some tips that will make sure you keep happily (and frequently) fed:

- In addition to packing healthy snacks, consider preparing some cold cereal and nonfat milk for yourself in the cap of a widemouthed thermos as a quick breakfast. Or buy a bagel and a piece of fruit, or a small carton of nonfat yogurt and some whole-grain bread and an apple. Stop off at a delicatessen for a little bit of cold chicken or turkey, or a can of water-packed tuna, and some whole-grain pita, fresh lettuce and tomatoes, and mustard for a good sandwich. Try for home-grown regional specialties—like peaches in Georgia, apples in Vermont, or oranges in Florida!
- If you've got the time and inclination, you might want to cook some of your own meals ahead and pack them in lightweight, portable plastic containers—perhaps a chick-pea salad, some cut-up cauliflower, peppers and cucumber with a curried mustard dip, along with some whole-grain muffins that might be hard to find on the road. One couple on the Pritikin program tells us they regularly pack an electric nonstick frying pan and small electric pot to prepare brown rice, oatmeal, and other cereals as well as soups—which they keep hot in a widemouthed thermos. This may sound a little ambitious, but it not only keeps them on track with their favorite foods, it saves them money as well!
- Ice chests are great for cold chicken, fresh vegetables, skim milk, prepared salads, sandwich spreads, and more—plus they give you the fun of a picnic wherever you go. They'll also enable you to store perishables as you travel, which you couldn't hang on to otherwise.

EATING OVERSEAS

Within America's relatively homogeneous culture (a coffee shop, a steak house, or certainly a fast-food place will be pretty much the same whether it's in New York, Oshkosh, Nashville, Los Angeles, or Chicago), you can already see that if you can take the Lifetime Eating Plan on the road in your hometown, there's no reason you can't take it several hundred miles away, too. Familiar foods are always available. But what happens when you leave the country? Is healthy eating impossible?

Healthy eating is *never* impossible—and it's usually very enjoyable—even when you're in an unfamiliar country. When you travel abroad, you'll often have plenty of native dishes to choose from that conform ideally to Pritikin plan guidelines; sometimes, as in the case of couscous or pasta dishes or the freshly baked whole-wheat breads available in European bakeries, it's even *easier* to eat healthy foods abroad than it is in our sometimes overprocessed country. If you can't avoid sampling a fatty native dish, then be sure you do just "sample" it. (You *can* experience a new food without overdoing it.)

You will, of course, have to make certain adjustments. The typical European continental breakfast features croissants, rolls, butter, and jam—and larger breakfasts feature meats and cheese, too. Limit yourself to the rolls and jam, and hot water for the herb tea you'll have brought along (or simply have hot water with lemon, which makes a refreshing hot drink, too). Hard-boiled eggs, fruit, and yogurt are also commonly available: Stick to the egg whites and fruit, and, if it's nonfat, the yogurt. (Obviously, if there's no alternative, you might choose low-fat yogurt, a "caution" food.) Also look in local markets for fresh produce or other healthy foods you can stock up on for the following morning's breakfast.

In fact, creating your own meals from local markets is a wonderful way of living like the natives do; it's not only the source of healthy alternatives, it can add to your traveling pleasure. Try making your own lunch from the specialties of the country—because some foods aren't or can't be exported, you'll taste fruits and vegetables and breads you literally can't get in the United States. In France, remove the *"croûte"* (or crust) from a dish like poached salmon *en croûte* and eat the unadorned fish; in Switzerland, eat only the boiled potatoes which the Swiss serve with shaved cheese in a national dish called *raclette*. One graduate student traveling in Italy was delighted to find he could indulge in some wonderful, imaginatively topped pizzas—the kinds *not* topped by cheese! Potatoes, onions, grilled eggplant, tuna, and artichokes were all alternatives on pizza, and they gave him some great ideas about how to prepare pizza when he got home.

When you're eating in restaurants for lunch or dinner abroad, follow the same restaurant tactics we outlined in Chapter 14. Of course, if you know the language well enough, you can try having your meals custom-cooked—which may turn out to be easier than doing it in the United States!

Dining in Tongues

With the help of Table 15-1 (see p. 292), next time you go abroad you can avoid the mystery dishes by ordering food custom-cooked to suit you. And don't worry if you haven't mastered the pronunciation—practicing some of these phrases ahead of time will make it easier to order in a new language.

DINNER PARTIES AND HOLIDAY MEALS

Back at home, you're eating happily and well on the Lifetime Eating Plan. But suddenly you take a look at the calendar: Only forty-five days left until Christmas! Could the July 4th family reunion picnic be coming up *that* soon? Oh, no—Easter, Labor Day, Thanksgiving, Hanukkah! You have visions (depending on the holiday) of stuffed turkeys or fried chicken, ice cream or holiday cakes and puddings, eggnogs and cases of cold beer—foods so completely associated with whatever the holiday is that you can't imagine celebrating without them.

Holidays (especially holidays that require your presence at other people's houses and parties) can sometimes be as stressful as they are delightful. Food is such an important part of these celebrations, and it's natural to be nervous. You're sure you'll hurt Grandma's feelings if you turn down her roast or her pie, and that Mom and Dad won't understand if you pass up the eggnog this year. You're also sure you'll feel deprived! At business or social holiday parties where the alcohol flows and high-fat canapés cover every table, how can you say no?

The Pritikin plan, as always, offers you alternatives—and, as usual, the alternatives will rarely make you feel you're depriving yourself. We say "rarely" because if you're obsessed with mincemeat pie with hard sauce and, fists clenched, decide not to have it at the last minute, then, yes, you'll feel deprived. But if you maintain a positive attitude, telling yourself that you don't need to eat unhealthy food to enjoy the holiday (and, in fact, can *increase* your enjoyment by sticking to nutritious fare), the cravings will pass. Take another look at the recipes in Chapter 13: You won't be stuck with celery stalks and tepid water while everyone else digs in. On the Pritikin plan, *you* can

TABLE 15-1
FOOD PHRASES IN TRANSLATION

English	Spanish	German	French	Italian
I must follow a special diet.	Yo debo seguir una dieta especial.	Ich muss eine besondere Diät einthalten.	Je dois suivre un régime spécial.	Devo seguire una dieta speciale.
All my food must be fat-free.	Es necessario que mi comida no tenga grasa.	Mein Essen darf kein Fett enthalten.	Tout doit être préparé sans gras.	Tutto dev' essere senza grassi.
Nothing can be fried.	No se debe freir nada.	Nichts darf gebraten werden.	Rien ne peut être frit.	Niente puo essere fritto.
please	por favor	bitte	s'il vous plaît	prego
thank you	gracias	danke	merci	grazie
baked	asado (for meat)	gebacken	au four	al forno
broiled	a la parrilla	im Ofen gebraten	grillé	al griglia
steamed	al vapor	gedämpft	à la vapeur	cotto a vapore
without	sin	ohne	sans	senza
sauce	salsa	Sauce	sauce	salsa
butter	mantequilla	Butter	beurre	burro
oil	aceite	Öl	huile	olio
cheese	queso	Käse	fromage	formaggio
salt	sal	Salz	sel	sale
sugar	azúcar	Zucker	sucre	zucchero
vegetables	legumbres	Gemüse	légumes	ortaggio, or legumi
salad	ensalada	Salat	salade	insalata
chicken	pollo	Hühnchen	poulet	pollo
fish	pescado	Fisch	poisson	pesce
beef	carne	Rindfleisch	boeuf	bue, or manzo

eat festively, too—you'll simply be giving yourself the added dividend of good health!

Now for some concrete suggestions. The wonderful new ideas you've already put to work in your daily life can be applied to holidays and special parties, too. You can enjoy your holidays in *every* way by celebrating with your mind and heart, as well as with great food. You'll have a great time eating—we promise you. Here are some tips:

- If you'll be attending a sit-down dinner and the host is a good friend, make your eating preferences known ahead of time so you can be better accommodated—perhaps with a special sauce or salad dressing the host will be happy to arrange for you. Most people will gladly help a friend who's attempting to stick to a healthy food regimen, particularly when the food preparation is so simple, as it is on the Pritikin plan.
- If you're really worried that you won't be able to resist the tempting food at a party or social event, snack before leaving home to take the edge off your hunger. Also, learn to decide whether you really are hungry—or if it's just nerves that makes you nibble on peanuts. At the party, sip a nonalcoholic beverage slowly; a carbonated mineral water, for example, will give you a nice feeling of satiety.
- As in restaurants, it's not a sin at a social gathering to politely but firmly refuse foods you don't want to eat. You don't have to resort to long-winded explanations, excuses, or apologies to pass up offers of inappropriate food. A simple "No, thanks, I'm doing fine" and a smile should satisfy your host at any occasion. (Remember, the host usually has a lot more on his or her mind than whether you're eating the canapés!) Feel free, on the other hand, to eat plentifully of the foods that *are* good for you.

IF YOU'RE THE HOST

You've got an advantage if you're the one giving the party—*you* get to plan what everybody eats! But how can you make sure they'll be satisfied with what they get? Here are a few suggestions from some veterans:

- Make some of the delicious, special entrees and desserts featured in Chapter 13: Chances are your guests will be enthusiastic (or at least curious) about trying and testing them out with you. The Cranberry-Glazed Chicken Breast with Whole-Grain Stuffing is a great guest pleaser (just increase the recipe accordingly).

- Offer your guests a choice of dishes or menus (for example, one for meat lovers and another for the grain-and-vegetable crowd) so they can be sure of having something they like.
- Potluck dinners are a fun way to solve the problem of pleasing everyone's palate. Try preparing the main entree, salad, and vegetable course (so you know you'll have a full, healthy meal for yourself) and have each person bring along a favorite food. By bringing your own dish to a potluck dinner, you'll have an opportunity to win converts, too!
- If you serve alcoholic beverages, do also offer alternatives like sparkling mineral water with ice and a squeeze of lemon, flavored seltzers, and nonalcoholic beer. If you choose to drink, combine your alcohol with seltzer, club soda (not high enough in sodium to present a problem for most people if drunk occasionally, although if you're salt sensitive, you'd do well to look for another alternative), vegetable juice, or fruit juice. Don't choose drinks that contribute fat, cholesterol, or sugar, such as a brandy alexander, eggnog, or Irish coffee. Whatever you drink, sip *slowly* and don't drink on an empty stomach: Always combine the beverage with food or have it after a meal. If you're curious about the calories in alcoholic beverages, Table 15-2 may be helpful.

STRESSLESS HOLIDAYS

During holiday time plan ahead so you can shop, bake, send cards, and entertain without being overly rushed, distracted, or fatigued. As we all know, holiday time can be full of pressure, and nervous tension and fatigue may influence you to make food choices you wouldn't make otherwise. Do be sure to exercise regularly; it will really help reduce excess stress. Set aside enough time to eat before shopping—heaven knows what you might bring home if you go to the market starving!—or carry some nutritious snacks with you. You'll keep your blood sugar and energy levels up, and be better able to meet holiday demands.

By pacing yourself, you'll avoid the last-minute flurry of activity that can send stress levels soaring. There's no reason that your regular eating schedule or routine of aerobic exercise and "rest peri-

TABLE 15-2
ALCOHOLIC BEVERAGE CALORIE COUNTER

Beverage	Serving Size (oz.)	Approximate Calories per Serving
Beer		
Regular	12	150
Light	12	100
Liquor, distilled spirits, 86 proof (gin, rum, vodka, whisky, scotch)	1.5	105
Wine		
Red or rosé	4	85
Dry white	4	80
Champagne	4	84
Appetizer/dessert		
Sherry	2	84
Port	2	90
Mixed drinks		
Bloody Mary	5	125
Martini	2.25	140
Manhattan	2.25	145
Whiskey sour	2.25	125
Old-fashioned	2.25	160
Tom Collins	10	180
Gin & tonic	8	185
Rum & coke	8	190
Screwdriver	8	200
Nonalcoholic beverages		
Seltzer, water	8	0
Juice spritzer	8	50–60

ods" has to change just because the holidays are coming up. In fact, if you've been pacing yourself all along, you may find you have more than enough time to meet any extra demands.

Above all, whatever the special event—whether it's a holiday party, or a trip abroad, or a business jaunt—enjoy yourself! Keep your sense of humor, and have fun with the people around you. Food is always a delightful part of celebrating, but it's not the only part: Atmosphere, the sights, any number of pleasures are available to you in addition to what's on your plate. You *can* enjoy eating healthfully anywhere—30,000 feet in the air or at your family's New Year's Eve party. There's no event, party, or place to which you can't bring the Pritikin plan—so have a delicious time of it!

CHAPTER 16

Moving Along and Feeling Great: Your Personalized Exercise Program

Want a perfect complement to the Pritikin Lifetime Eating Plan, and another *enjoyable* way to get rid of excess pounds? Exercise. How about a surefire remedy for fatigue and stiffness, or the stresses of the daily grind? Try exercise! Want to build up your cardiovascular strength, lower your blood pressure, and have a good time doing it? You guessed it—the right exercise program, in combination with a sound diet, will do it all (and more), and leave you feeling fabulous, too.

If exercising regularly is one of the most wonderful things we can do for ourselves, why do so many of us say "This is not for me"? Well, if you haven't exercised since school gym (ten, twenty, thirty, or more years ago), the idea of duplicating or even approximating what you did as a youth *can* be intimidating. All those jumping jacks, push-ups, sit-ups, laps around the track—the very thought is unappealing. You may also feel a bit of secret embarrassment at how you think you'd *look* now in the gym, on the track, or in the park. "How could I possibly measure up to those lithe, youthful runners I see passing me by? It's all pretty much out of the question now—isn't it?"

297

No! If you did it before—or even if you didn't—you can probably do it now.

If we succeed at all at the Pritikin Centers in getting people who've never exercised to start a regular exercise program (and we do), it's because of this simple exercise advice: Keep your activities simple, convenient, and enjoyable! And don't go on the (dangerous) presumption that you have to work out as hard and as fast as you may have done at eighteen. Believe it or not, you can fashion a safe, highly effective program around one of the most pleasant activities we know—walking. In fact, any amount of aerobic exercise appears to provide some benefit. In one study, those who exercised enough to burn in excess of 2,000 calories per week reduced their risk of heart attack by 36 percent.[1] So a brisk one-hour walk every day can have *real* cardiovascular benefit. Of course, some people may make dramatic progress from this modest beginning. Perhaps the most moving examples of this are the numerous people who've come to Pritikin Centers suffering from such severe claudication (atherosclerosis in the legs causing sometimes debilitating pain) that they could barely walk across the room, much less around the block. Within weeks, these people were walking half a mile; within months, a mile, two miles, or more. One went on to run a marathon!

The benefits of regular exercise are considerable and numerous—and research continues to turn up more. A consistent, personally tailored exercise program will enhance your cardiovascular fitness, help you burn extra calories, boost your everyday endurance, lessen fatigue, help you sleep better, and increase your overall strength and flexibility. What's more, you'll enjoy lower blood pressure, quicker recovery of the pulse following exercise, bowel regularity, improved muscle tone, an improved HDL ("good") cholesterol level, improved glucose metabolism, and lower blood levels of triglycerides. *Over*-exercising is, however, bad news. It not only increases the risk of physical injury, but it turns what has the potential of being enjoyable, energizing activity into a dreaded chore. You wouldn't want to stick with an eating plan you don't enjoy—why should exercise be any different? Focus on the benefits of exercise *and* on doing the activities you enjoy, in the way that's right for you. Knowing your exercise program is manageable and fun will encourage you to make it a regular part of your life!

WHAT IS AEROBIC EXERCISE?

You've undoubtedly heard of the two categories of exercise: aerobic and anaerobic. The first—aerobic—is what we want you to do, or at least concentrate on most. Why? Aerobic (which literally means "with oxygen") exercise conditions your heart, lungs, and circulatory system—it's the exercise that makes and keeps you "fit." Some good examples are brisk walking, jogging, lap swimming, cycling, cross-country skiing, and aerobic dancing.

In order to perform their various functions, our muscles need a constant supply of oxygen, which is provided by the blood our heart pumps throughout our system. Every heartbeat sends another "shot" of this valuable fuel throughout the body, and especially to those places where the body is working the hardest. Not surprisingly, the more oxygen we are able to utilize in our muscles, the more easily and longer they can do their routine work—and the better we feel.

In an aerobic workout, the body's large muscles move in a continuous, rhythmic manner. The demand for oxygen to fuel those muscles is great, so the heart responds by pumping blood at a faster rate, sending out a greater supply of oxygen and keeping it readily available so the exercise can be sustained over a long period of time. (Aerobic exercise is effective for cardiovascular health only when it elevates the heart rate for at least 20 consecutive minutes at a time.) This heightened pumping activity is the heart's response to the demand of the workout, and thereby strengthens the heart, empowering it to work more efficiently and more healthfully on a day-to-day basis by pumping *more* blood in *fewer*, but stronger, beats.

By contrast, anaerobic ("without oxygen") exercise, like sprinting or power-lifting, is performed for a much shorter time at a higher level of intensity. You become "winded" quite easily because your circulatory system can't supply adequate oxygen for your muscles' needs during the intense burst of activity. The recent emphasis on joining a gym to lift weights or work out on machines like the Nautilus has attracted a lot of people to this kind of working out. It's important to understand that while anaerobic exercises can build up muscles, they do little or nothing at all for cardiovascular fitness. (Although there *is* a way to work out with weights or on machines that helps aerobically, called "circuit training," it's not what many people turn to weights to do.) You may feel as if you've had quite a workout after lifting weights, but unless you're doing it aerobically, you aren't strengthening your heart.

Another misconception about anaerobic exercise is that it will help you lose fat. Actually, you burn very few calories in anaerobic exercise, as compared to aerobic—you simply can't keep up the activity long enough to burn a significant number of calories. You'll strengthen your muscles, but if, for example, you're worried about your "spare tire," the most that anaerobic sit-ups or abdominal crunches on the Nautilus can do is make it a steel-belted radial! You may firm up some muscle, but the padding of fat won't diminish appreciably. Moreover, working out with weights can actually be dangerous for some people—the sudden intense effort can raise blood pressure and increase the risk of stroke.

However, weight training can be used aerobically to gain strength or as a regular addition to aerobic exercise if you're cleared medically to do it. Anaerobic exercise doesn't have to be bad for you; it's just that the right aerobic exercise is much easier, and *so* much better for your cardiovascular health. And remember, it can begin with, and remain, something as simple as walking!

AEROBIC EXERCISE: A BOOST TO WEIGHT LOSS

While it *is* possible to "sweat away" a few pounds, the weight you lose from sweating is only water. But exercise does, of course, help you lose what you *want* to lose—fat. We've emphasized the cardiovascular benefits of exercise because they're so considerable, but the bonus benefit is that, if you're overweight, consistent aerobic exercise will help you lose that weight. In fact, if you find yourself stuck at a certain weight, exercise can help push you over the temporary hurdle by increasing your metabolic rate and lowering your "setpoint"— the weight your body itself tries to maintain once you lose excess pounds.

Remember, we recommend that you do not consume fewer than 1,000 calories a day if you're a woman or 1,200 calories if you're a man—because fewer calories than those levels will sacrifice lean muscle as well as fat, and can hamper your efforts to keep off the weight you lose. Aerobic exercise produces exactly the opposite effect: It helps you burn more calories and possibly build lean body mass while eliminating surplus fat.

Because muscle tissue weighs more than fat, you may not see any dramatic difference on the scale at first—but you will if you use a tape measure! The new taut muscle has less volume, which means your body shape will definitely change for the better—perhaps by as much as several clothing sizes—before you know it. Your waist, abdomen, hips, thighs—wherever fat accumulates so visibly—will now look leaner, firmer, and more shapely and defined. Even if your weight stays the same on the scale, you can still achieve a significant reduction in your body-fat percentage. Thus, if you're a woman whose weight remains at 135 pounds but is now only 24 percent fat (and more muscle) instead of 30 percent fat, you will no longer be "overfat." This is why we've been stressing losing fat rather than weight, and why scales can be so misleading. Any additional muscle mass will actually assist in burning more calories!

Muscle is a more metabolically active tissue than fat: It demands more of the body's energy to keep it going and so is "hungrier" for calories, using them up more readily. Obviously, the more of this lean tissue you have, the easier it will be to lose weight. Another bit of good news: The increased metabolic effect of aerobic exercise carries over for about three hours. You'll burn more calories *after* exercising—even at rest—than you would if you hadn't exercised.

BEFORE YOU BEGIN

According to the American College of Sports Medicine (ACSM), if you are an apparently healthy adult under age forty-five without any known risk factors for coronary disease, you can usually start an exercise program without the need for prior medical screening, as long as you begin and proceed very gradually and are alert to the development of any unusual symptoms.[2] But underscore *healthy:* If you have (or suspect you may have) even one major risk factor for heart disease (high blood pressure, diabetes, elevated cholesterol, etc.), or if you have a diagnosed illness, you should not proceed on any exercise program without first consulting your doctor. And you should call your doctor if you're over forty-five, whatever the state of your health. This is crucial not only because it makes good sense, but also because plunging yourself into a strenuous exercise regimen (like jogging) can be dangerous, even life-threatening, if you're at risk for heart disease. Even the healthiest-looking people can discover, to their dismay, that their arteries are clogged and their blood pressure is dangerously high. But they would never have known if they hadn't sought medical advice.

Since you don't have to show symptoms of cardiovascular disease to have it, think carefully about what exercise is best for you. For many heart-disease victims, the *first* symptom is sudden death! Abruptly starting an overly strenuous exercise routine can cause severe stress to your heart. So if there's any doubt about your cardiovascular health when you start to exercise, *don't* go for something strenuous like jogging—try walking instead. More important, see your doctor first.

The point is to find an activity that's safe for you and that you enjoy doing, and to do it in a way which will make it optimally beneficial. Your doctor can help you sort this out, perhaps on the basis of a complete treadmill stress test (this makes particularly good sense if you want to exercise vigorously) and a blood test to determine your cholesterol, triglyceride, and glucose values. If you're over forty-five and at risk for heart and lung disease, it's even more important that your doctor administer these tests before you embark on any exercise program at all.

That said, let's return to a promise we made at the outset: There is nothing more enjoyable than following a *safe*, regular program of exercise. Once you choose the right exercise for you—and learn to do it within the safe range of your "THR" (that's your training, or target, heart rate, which we'll explain next)—we can virtually guarantee you won't want to stop!

SOME IMPORTANT EXERCISE REMINDERS

- If you're over forty-five, see your doctor before you begin *any* exercise program.
- Select aerobic activities.
- Build up your exercise program gradually.
- Plan to work out regularly.

HOW TO GET F.I.T.

So many people have come to our Pritikin Longevity Centers convinced they could never run, walk, jog, swim, row, cycle, or dance. So many of the same people now (you guessed it) run, walk, jog, swim, row, cycle, and dance! The most joyous thing about exercise is the one that can't be conveyed in writing—the *feeling* you get when you do it regularly, and for a long enough session that it benefits you aerobically. It's not only a feeling of accomplishment (which is, of course, considerable)—you get a physical "lift" that lasts for the whole day.

Once you know it's safe to begin an exercise program, how hard should you exercise, and how often? The recommendation is to work out continuously at your training heart rate for at least 20 minutes three times a week, and at least once a week just below your THR. To help you with your program, we've developed a personal workout plan that consists of three main variables: frequency, intensity, and time—easily remembered as "F.I.T."

Frequency

How often you exercise is one factor in generating the results you're looking for in an exercise program. We recommend four to six aerobic workouts a week. That may be difficult, but try not to skip two days of exercise in a row—it can be hard to get back on track when you do. There's also the possibility that your level of triglycerides (circulating blood fats), which is sharply reduced by aerobic exercise, may promptly increase in its absence.

Intensity

This measure is determined by your training (or target) heart rate—your THR. It's important that your heart stay within this range for you to get optimal cardiovascular benefit; anything less won't give you full benefit, and going above your range will quickly render your exercise anaerobic (not oxygen-efficient), and could be dangerous as well. A general rule is that if you can speak or hum easily while you exercise, you're not overdoing it. Heavy breathing is okay, but gasping for breath is not, since it might mean you're not getting enough oxygen. So at the first sign of dizziness or shortness of breath, *slow down*, and then stop—especially if you know you're at risk for heart disease. Although it's hard for most people to keep exercising above their THR, a feeling of light-headedness can be a sign that you *are*—which could lead to an increased risk of injury, an elevation in your blood pressure, or the precipitation of arrhythmia (an alteration in the rhythm of the heartbeat) or ischemia (obstruction of the inflow of arterial blood).

The most accurate way to determine your training heart rate is to take a treadmill test—and for some people, as we mentioned earlier, it's the *only* safe way. But if you're ready to begin exercising (according to the ACSM guidelines cited earlier) you can simply calculate your general training heart rate. The following formula is, however, *not* appropriate (and can even be dangerous) for people with some medical conditions (such as high blood pressure) or for those taking certain medications (such as a beta-blocker). Calculating your own THR is appropriate *only* for those who are not at risk.

Calculating your THR. First, subtract your age from 220 (everyone's base number). Multiply the result by .7 to find the lower limit of your THR, and then by .85 to determine the upper limit. These numbers are your training heart rate *range*, per minute. However, if you stop to check your heart rate during a workout, don't take your pulse for a full minute—by the time the 60 seconds are up, your heart rate will have gone way down. Take it for a shorter period of time, then multiply the reading to equal a full minute. Many regular exercisers find it easiest just to multiply a 6-second reading by 10 to find out if they're on target.

For example, if you're 35:

220 (everyone's base number)
− 35 (age)
185 (age-predicted maximum heart rate)

185	185
× .70	× .85
129.50	157.25

(low limit of training   (high limit of training
heart rate,   heart rate,
per minute)   per minute)

129–157 is your THR range, per minute.

To take your pulse, use the index and middle fingers of one hand to find your pulse under your thumb on the wrist of the opposite hand. (Some people find it easier to place the index and middle fingers of one hand on their upper neck, right below their jaw, to find their pulse. Either way is fine—just don't press too hard, and don't press on both sides of the neck at once.)

Practice taking your pulse regularly when you exercise to see if you're on target, and try to be conscious of what your body feels like when you're within range. Most people describe this feeling as exertion just above what's easy—when they're conscious of the exertion but can hum or talk easily to a companion, and feel as though they could keep moving for a fairly long time. (Runners often say they're there when their breathing "kicks in." And for some people, it's their "sweat threshold"—but don't count on that as a perfect indicator, since heat, humidity, and individual metabolism make people sweat at different times.) Do try to sensitize yourself to what your THR feels like *inside;* after a while, you won't need to keep checking your pulse—you'll just have a gut feeling that you're on track.

Hard and easy days. The "I" of F.I.T.—intensity—also has to do with hard and easy exercising days: Our recommendation is that you alternate between them. On a "hard" day, perform any aerobic workout at your training heart rate for a maximum advantage to your heart and lungs. On "easy" days, do the same activity but at 4 to 12 beats (per 60-second count) below your training heart rate, and for a longer duration than on a "hard" day. Exercising both "hard" and "easy" will not only develop your endurance and help you burn fat, but it will also reduce your chances of being injured by overtraining by allowing your body time to adapt (on easy days) to the stress of exercise.

You'll find that the more fit you become, the more "work" it takes to achieve and maintain your THR: You'll probably have to step up the rate of whatever exercise you're doing. But don't worry—you'll be ready. You'll be more fit, and you'll probably *want* to move a little more by that time as well, exercising most days at your THR.

Time

On hard days, exercise for 30 to 45 minutes at training heart rate; on easy days, exercise for 45 to 60 minutes below your THR, as described above. This is only a general rule, however; if you're just starting an exercise program, simply do the best you can and aim for 20 minutes at first on both hard and easy days. Extend your exercise sessions gradually as your fitness improves, until you reach the recommended lengths of time. Some people may be able to do this quite easily—but be careful not to overdo it! It just isn't necessary (and may be unwise) to log in excessive amounts of time.

If you choose to walk or jog, you might want to wear a pedometer to gauge your distance. Or drive your car along your course to check the mileage. (You can even figure out your walking or running rate if you divide your distance by your time. If, for example, it takes you 24 minutes to run a 2-mile course—including a 3-minute walking break between the first and second miles—divide the 21 minutes you run by the 2 miles you cover. You're running a $10\frac{1}{2}$-minute mile.)

WARMING UP

Whatever shape you're in, you need to warm up. A good warm-up will stretch your muscles, dilate your blood vessels, and step up your heart rate gradually. By increasing the muscles' blood supply and raising their temperature, warming up makes them more flexible and less prone to pulls and strains. Warming up will help prevent injuries and soreness, as well as sudden cardiovascular stress. It will also improve your coordination and enhance your range of motion.

If you're anxious to get going, you may be tempted to skip your warm-up, but remember: Even the most superbly conditioned athletes need to warm up before they exercise—and pay a price if they don't. (One experienced athlete thought she'd try "just this once" playing a fast game of tennis without warming up—and ended up with a torn muscle.)

Your warm-up involves doing your chosen exercise, but at a slower pace; this will give your heart a sufficient supply of blood so it can meet its increased demand for oxygen during the workout to follow. How long should you do this? A minimum of 5 minutes is usually fine, but if you have a heart condition, hypertension, or claudication, take 7 to 10 minutes in warm weather and an additional 5 minutes in cold weather. Everyone should take longer to warm up in cold weather—a minimum of 10 minutes. Regardless of how fit you are, remember: The warm-up is essential. Stress tests have shown that even the best-conditioned athletes may have irregular heartbeats if they skip warming up—as well as put themselves at risk of muscle or tendon injury.

COOLING DOWN

Just as a plane takes off, spends most of its time soaring at a certain altitude, and then has to be brought carefully down, so you have to come "down" from your workout with care. A cool-down is a sort of reverse warm-up. Ending your workout too abruptly may cause your heart rate and blood pressure to become erratic and your blood to pool in the muscles of your legs and arms. With less blood available for the brain and heart, you may feel dizzy or faint, and experience irregular heartbeats. (You should *not* be in great pain the day after a workout—if you are, it means you've either overdone it or performed an exercise incorrectly.)

To cool down, walk slowly and continuously for about 5 minutes; this will maintain the normal circulation you need to prevent the pooling effect, and will flush away lactic acid. In hot, humid weather, increase the length of your cool-down by another 5 minutes to help your body return to normal resting levels. Check your pulse rate, too, after 5 minutes of cooling down: If you're still within your THR range, continue to cool down for a couple of minutes more until your pulse rate drops beneath the lower number of your training range. (When you stop to take your pulse, be sure to keep your hips and legs "swaying" so that your contracting muscles assist in moving blood back to your heart.)

To prevent dehydration, always drink plenty of fluids after your workout (particularly in very cold or hot weather). Drink 6 to 8 ounces of fluid before you work out and then sip some fluid every 15 to 20 minutes during your workout as well. Avoid sugary, caffeinated, and alcoholic drinks, as you always would. And be sure to wait at least 15 to 20 minutes after your cool-down to shower or bathe, or to get into a whirlpool or sauna. This will give your body time to bring its core temperature back to normal. If you have health concerns, check with your physician before using a Jacuzzi or sauna.

STRETCHING

Regular stretching will promote circulation, reduce muscle tension, improve coordination, and help prevent injuries. The best time to do stretching exercises is after you've cooled down—you especially need to stretch your calves and hamstrings. Muscles benefit more by being stretched after they have been warmed up and exercised: Warmer muscles are more pliable and therefore more easily stretched, and movement increases blood flow to the muscles, thereby increasing the muscle temperature.

HAMSTRING STRETCH

Place one foot on a low support in front of you. Bend from the hips, keeping your back straight. Press hand on thigh until you feel a stretch in the back of the thigh and behind the knee.

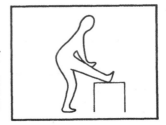

SHIN AND CALF STRETCH

Flex and point foot and make circles with the ankle. This stretch is helpful in preventing shinsplints.

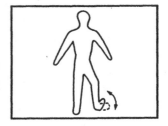

CALF STRETCH

a. Begin by standing and facing a wall. Place hands on the wall at shoulder height and width. Keep your back straight.
b. Place right food forward, left foot back (keep toes pointing straight ahead).
c. Shift weight onto left leg, keeping heel on the floor. Lean toward the wall to increase

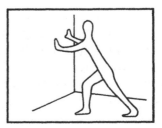

stretch. Go only to the point of resistance, then hold for 10 to 15 seconds.

d. Change legs. Repeat 2 times for each leg.

ACHILLES-TENDON STRETCH

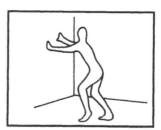

a. Begin by standing and facing a wall. Place hands on the wall at shoulder height and width. Keep back straight.
b. Place left foot foward, right foot back.
c. Bend knees slightly, keeping heels on ground.
d. Feel the stretch near the back heel. Hold for 10 to 15 seconds.
e. Repeat on other leg.

WHAT ARE YOUR EXERCISE OPTIONS?

As you'll soon see, there are many aerobic options to choose from, even if you haven't exercised in years. Our favorite, of course, is walking—and what a revelation it can be to take a healthful walk! Keeping up your stride at the right degree of intensity, for the right amount of time, can soon become second nature, and it will allow you to see and appreciate your surroundings while providing you all the benefits of aerobic exercise.

Because it's so easy and so popular (95 percent of Pritikin Center alumni choose walking as their exercise), as well as one of the best and safest exercises you can choose, we'll start our list of exercises with walking. But read through the *whole* list. As much as consistency is important in an exercise routine, variety can help to keep your interest and enjoyment high. You may want to use a stationary cycle or a rowing machine as well as walk—or roller-skate, swim, or dance aerobically. Don't, however, expect that the average game of squash, racquetball, or tennis will give you the same benefit. Sports such as these don't qualify as aerobic workouts unless you're a superb athlete who keeps moving throughout the whole 30-, 45-, or 60-minute period—difficult to do, even for the most experienced player. You want to maintain your movement (and thus a *constant* training heart rate), which generally means taking part in one or more of the following exercises.

Walking

The right kind of walking will give you top aerobic benefits. Don't think that because it looks easier than running it's not terrific exercise—it is! Just think about it: With every step you're lifting your body weight. Walking will firm up and define the gluteal muscles in your buttocks, the muscles in your calves, your quadriceps (front thigh muscles), and, to a lesser degree, your hamstrings. The best thing about walking, of course, is that everybody can do it. And except for a good pair of shoes and socks, walking requires no special equipment.

When you start, do so at a comfortable pace, then increase your speed and time gradually as your endurance builds up. Remember, a casual stroll—while it's a little better than no exercise at all—will not help you achieve your training heart rate or provide you with optimal aerobic benefits. But once you're moving along at the rate that's right for you, you will improve both your health *and* your chances of successful weight loss. Walking is a safe, easy, and enjoyable way to keep fit. It's such a natural that you'll want to make it a mainstay of your exercise regimen.

Jogging

If you want to jog and your physician approves (if you have arthritis it may not be a good idea, or if you're more than 20 pounds overweight running may be unduly stressful to your ankles, knees, and hips), you'll get exercise benefits faster than from walking, but remember to start out slowly and build up speed only as your fitness increases. (If you're overweight, you'll find your pace picking up as you lose weight.) Proper warm-up and cool-down sessions (see pages 306–307) are critical; the calf, hamstring, and Achilles-tendon stretching exercises illustrated on pages 308–309 are especially important before and after jogging to prevent muscle pulls and strains.

If you haven't exercised regularly for the past three months or more, don't push yourself, even if your doctor says jogging would be all right for you. Start with a walking program for the first few weeks to minimize wear and tear on your muscles and get your body used to moving at a steady rate and intensity. Then, when you feel you're ready, step up your pace to a slow jog (after a good walking warm-up) and maintain the jog as long as it's comfortable. Drop back to a walk for as many minutes as you feel you need, then jog again when you're ready. Gradually you can work up to longer, more vigorous jogging sessions.

The easiest and best way to know the correct speed for you is to check your pulse rate. Exert yourself until you feel your heart beating faster and until you've reached your training heart rate—but don't go over that rate. Check your pulse as often as you need to (sway your hips while you do, so your blood won't pool in your arm or leg muscles). If you're short of breath or unable to talk, you're working too hard: Slow down, perhaps to a walk. If you're not jogging with a companion, try humming or singing to yourself; you're not overdoing it if you can still speak easily. Or just sing along with a tape! (Many people find running to music keeps them going longer and farther, as well.)

Bicycling

Biking can offer an excellent aerobic workout, especially in hilly areas. If you're a beginner, the low gears on a 10- or 12-speed bicycle can help you negotiate even the steepest hills until you are conditioned enough to climb them in higher gears. To avoid sore knees, make sure your bicycle seat is neither too high nor too low. An easy test: Sit on your bicycle, and with the ball of your right foot push the right pedal around and down as far as it will go. If your knee is just slightly flexed—not locked straight—the seat is probably just right. When you ride, keep the balls of your feet on the pedals. Also, to avoid knee strain, select gears that are easy to ride in. Forcing too hard with high gears creates strain.

As with jogging, if you haven't exercised regularly for a long time, don't start cycling right away. While walking makes daily use of the muscles in the back of the thigh (the hamstrings), both outdoor and stationary cycling work the less-utilized quadriceps in the front of the thigh. Outdoor riding on even a moderately hilly terrain will give you a good challenge, but until your "quads" are trained and you can pedal "against resistance" for at least 30 minutes, it's best to rely on walking or jogging as your primary form of exercise. Or if you have an indoor cycle which adjusts for varying levels of resistance (most do), or a device to turn your 10- or 12-speed bicycle into an exercise cycle, set the resistance or the gears on low and maintain a constant speed. Then step up both the gears and your speed as your leg strength increases with practice. Check your pulse from time to time to make sure you haven't "coasted" out of your training heart rate range.

The benefits of cycling—whether on a stationary bike or outdoors—are improved cardiovascular function, enhanced muscle tone, and definition in your legs. (This will be most noticeable on your quadriceps, but you'll also see some change on your hamstrings and a bit on your calves.) If you want more of an upper-body workout, look for a stationary bicycle such as a Schwinn Air-Dyne, which provides for arm movement as well.

Warm-up and cool-down sessions are as important to cyclists as they are to joggers and runners; be sure to include stretches for all your leg muscles after a bicycling workout. Outdoor cyclists should heed this winter warning, too: Take greater precautions against frostbite than joggers would because of the wind you generate while riding, even on calm or not terribly cold days.

Swimming

If you have the strength and skill, continuous lap swimming in the crawl or breaststroke can be an ideal exercise since it conditions several muscle groups and works the heart and lungs without any harmful impact on muscles, tendons, or bones. And the benefits of regular swimming are aesthetic as well as healthful: In addition to providing excellent cardiovascular conditioning, swimming develops muscles in the chest, arms, shoulders, and legs to give you very well-balanced proportions.

If you don't yet swim well enough for an extended workout, consider taking lessons to improve your technique, and supplement your time in the pool with regular walking or other aerobic exercise. It's not as easy as it may seem to make swimming an effective aerobic workout if you're simply used to taking the occasional dip in the pool, lake, or ocean: As with any exercise, to be aerobically effective it must be kept up for the right amount of time and at the right intensity. So if you need practice, lessons, or just a place to swim, check with your local YMCA or YWCA, health clubs, community colleges, and municipal recreation areas for information on pools, instruction, and endurance swim programs.

Like walking, jogging, and cycling, swimming requires warm-ups and cool-downs. Be sure to follow the warming-up, cooling-down, and stretching advice outlined on pages 306–309.

MORE EXERCISE IDEAS

Other terrific aerobic exercises include cross-country skiing (either outdoors or on an indoor cross-country skiing machine), working out on a rowing machine, or using a treadmill (it may take some practice before you're proficient enough to do it at the right intensity and for the right amount of time, so be patient!). Or you might enjoy using such relatively unusual stationary bicycles as a Schwinn Air-Dyne, which incorporates arm movement, or even a "recumbent" bike, which permits you to cycle in a horizontal position (great for reading!)

Rowing demands that your back and knees be in reasonably good condition, and technique is very important, too. You can usually get access to a treadmill through a health club or a gym, although you may want to consider purchasing a treadmill, since it's such a terrific exercise device: It allows you to walk at varying speeds and grades without ever leaving home! The treadmill, in fact, is the exercise equipment we recommend for almost everyone at our Pritikin Centers.

Unless you have high blood pressure, you might want to walk with hand weights for a greater challenge. (If you do have high blood pressure, however, you should not—except under a doctor's supervision—indulge in any kind of upper-body exercise such as carrying hand weights, since it increases your blood pressure much more than it increases your heart rate.) If you want variety, you can do 10 minutes of one activity (walking on a treadmill, for example), 10 minutes of a second (pedaling on a stationary bike), and 10 minutes of a third (using the rowing machine). If you take this "alternate" approach, just be sure to move from one activity to the other as quickly as you can (while maintaining safety) so your heart rate doesn't have a chance to go down. You want to keep your training heart rate steady—but not go above it. We can't emphasize this enough: Don't overdo it!

As we mentioned before, you can also do a workout with weights or resistance machines for aerobic benefit—but you have to be in good shape to do this, so don't make that a priority if you're just beginning to exercise. And a reminder about sports like tennis, basketball, racquetball, and especially the less strenuous golf and bowling: These aren't aerobic conditioning exercises (unless, as we've said, you can keep them up at the right intensity for the right amount of time—which is impossible with a golf club or a bowling ball!). Tennis may not help aerobics, but aerobics *will* help your tennis—or whatever other recreational sport you decide to pursue.

Some people find it helpful to exercise with a friend. Working out with a companion sometimes gives you moral reinforcement and helps you keep your appointment to exercise. But don't skip an exercise session just because your friend wants to! And don't make your exercise program dependent on good weather; investigate opportunities at health clubs or indoor pools, gyms, and tracks at places like local schools—even shopping malls, as long as you don't stop to window-shop! Inclement weather doesn't have to keep you from working out. There are aerobic fitness or dance classes, even taped exercise sessions you can follow on your VCR. Just keep your eyes open—and your exercise shoes on!

USE EVERY OPPORTUNITY!

You can make exercise a part of your daily life more easily than you may think. How? By substituting an *active* way of getting things done for a sedentary way. The following hints should help:

- Use the stairs instead of the elevator.
- Don't take a bus at the stop nearest your home, but walk briskly to one 20 or 30 minutes away.
- Walk or ride your bicycle to work, to the market, or to do errands.
- Take exercise breaks instead of coffee breaks.
- Park your car at the far end of the lot and walk from there.

GEARING UP

If you plan to walk or jog, well-fitted shoes are a *must*. Tennis shoes or sneakers just won't do, because they don't have the proper support and cushioning to cradle the foot firmly and absorb shock. Look for shoes that feel lightweight and comfortable with one pair of good cotton socks. To prevent corns and blisters, make sure your shoes leave enough room for your toes at the front (about a thumb's width), since feet will swell slightly during exercise. A snug but not-too-tight feeling is best, not just around the toes but for the entire foot. A sturdy heel cup (to prevent slippage and friction blisters), good arch support, flexibility, and a well-cushioned sole are also essential. Bear in mind, too, that if the shoe is advertised as a "walking" shoe, that's what it should be used for—*not* for jogging.

What you wear (above the ankles) may range from shorts and a T-shirt in summer to several lightweight layers plus a hat and gloves in winter. Long johns under loose cotton exercise pants, a long-sleeved cotton T-shirt, and a sweater under a windbreaker are best for very cold days. Walkers or outdoor cyclists may want a light backpack to store extra layers of clothes to either shed or don as weather conditions (or degree of comfort) change. Many joggers find this uncomfortable, however, and simply tie an extra garment around their waist by the sleeves. (Winter bicyclists should dress more warmly than winter joggers, to compensate for the wind they create when really moving along.) A small "fanny-pack" is sometimes convenient for keys, money, or a hat and gloves.

Some people think they'll lose weight faster if they overdress or wear a nylon jogging or "condition" suit to sweat away extra pounds. But the only thing they'll sweat away is water—weight that starts coming back as soon as they drink their next glass of liquid. More critical, overdressing during vigorous exercise, just like working out too hard in hot, humid weather, can impede the normal evaporation of sweat, your body's natural cooling system, and increase your risk of heat stroke.

WHAT EXERCISE CAN'T DO

Aerobic exercise is fabulous: It boosts cardiovascular fitness by making the heart a highly efficient pump that delivers more blood and oxygen to all the body's tissues, especially muscle cells. It also lowers serum triglycerides (blood fats), blood pressure, and blood glucose; increases the size of coronary vessels; and builds the body's army of cholesterol-scavenging HDLs (high-density lipoproteins, or "good" cholesterol).

It's crucial to remember, however, that with all its benefits, aerobic exercise has at best limited effectiveness in protecting you from cardiovascular disease if it's not complemented by a healthy diet. Remember the marathon runners we spoke about who looked lithe and lean, but who were still at great risk of heart disease? Vigorous workouts won't significantly offset the effects of a high-cholesterol diet because, unlike fat, cholesterol, particularly LDL cholesterol, itself cannot be "burned" away. Again, the saddest and most dramatic illustrations of this fact are the long-distance runners who have died suddenly in their thirties, forties, and fifties—often while engaged in their sport.

The reason we're reemphasizing this is to counter the myth that it doesn't matter what you eat as long as you exercise: Believe us, it does! Despite their appearance and athletic feats, marathon runners who've suffered sudden fatal heart attacks have been found (in autopsies) to have severe clogging in their major coronary arteries. Aerobic exercise alone—even a lifetime of competitive running—will not grant you immunity from coronary artery disease. Only by making the right food choices can your risk be diminished and coronary disease be slowed, stopped, or reversed.

This is clear evidence for why we want you to follow a combined program of good food habits *and* exercise. Exercise can complement the right food plan dramatically, but it can never substitute for it. (Of course, if you follow a fatty, salty, high-cholesterol diet, you are surely better off exercising less strenuously than if you ate sensibly: The progressive artery-clogging effects of a poor eating plan are not compatible with a stressful, vigorous workout.)

And a good food plan will complement your exercise, too: The right foods will give you the energy you need for any vigorous physical activity. In fact, most people who eat meals low in fat and high in complex carbohydrates are able to work out longer before feeling fatigued than those on a high-fat, high-protein diet. Obviously, the Pritikin Lifetime Eating Plan fits the bill—it's ideally compatible with an active life!

EXERCISE QUESTIONS MOST COMMONLY ASKED

Here are a few questions about exercise that are frequently asked; you may be able to answer some of them already, based on what you've learned so far. (At least if someone asks you about the role of exercise in your life, or how and why you do it, you'll be prepared to clear up some myths!)

Q: *Why is a 20-minute workout better than two 10-minute workouts?*
A: Twenty continuous minutes is the minimum amount of time needed to produce a cardiovascular training effect.

Q: *If your training heart rate is a range, how do you determine where in the range to exercise?*
A: You can exercise so your heart rate is anywhere above the minimum, but the higher you are within your heart rate range, the better. Remember to monitor yourself so you don't go above the maximum rate.

Q: *Does walking help to firm up fat?*
A: You cannot "firm up" fat, but brisk walking does burn fat, and also helps to firm up muscles. Walking at your training heart rate will give you all the benefits of aerobic exercise.

Q: *Is there a certain amount of time you need to wait between exercise sessions?*
A: There is no set time you should wait between aerobic exercise sessions, but adequate rest ensures that workouts will be of high quality. Most exercisers work out once a day.

Q: *Should I stretch before or after I've worked out?*
A: Either is fine, but both is best. Stretching should be a part of your daily exercise program, and should also be done after your cool-down. Stretching before you work out prepares your muscles for exercise; however, you may get more of a stretch and potentially more benefit from a muscle that has been warmed by your workout.

Q: *Why can't I use my aerobic shoes for walking or running?*
A: Aerobic shoes are not designed for walking or running. The sole of an aerobic shoe is narrower and there isn't enough support. But the flared heel of a running shoe dissipates the force of running over the entire foot, and the wide sole provides better footing than an aerobic shoe.

Q: *How will I know when I've reached my training heart rate during exercise?*
A: The best way to keep track of your training heart rate is to stop and check your pulse. Do this quickly, because your heart rate will begin to drop shortly after you stop moving.

Q: *Why do I get out of breath when I exercise?*
A: That out-of-breath feeling is not generally due to a problem in the lungs, but rather is related to the inability of the heart to properly deliver enough blood and oxygen to the muscles. Remember not to exercise past the point where you can speak easily.

Q: *What happens if I drop my exercise program for a month?*
A: You may feel as if you are starting at square one again, since you lose fitness about twice as fast as you build it up. Remember, if you don't use it, you'll lose it—quickly.

Q: *What if I'm sick?*
A: It is better not to exercise if you're ill or have a fever or muscle aches, since your body is already under stress and additional stress could be harmful. After even a minor illness, you should resume your exercise

EXERCISE WHEN YOU TRAVEL

Wherever you travel and for whatever reason—business or pleasure—there's no need to leave exercise behind! In fact, exercising in a new place, on a different schedule, can be a refreshing break from your regular workout routine. Here are some tips that will show you how easy it can be to keep fit, even in transit:

- Get used to a variety of exercises, so if you find yourself away from home and unable to do what you like best, you'll be able to choose something else (for example, walking instead of biking).
- When you make your hotel reservations, inquire about exercise facilities. Hotels that don't have their own facilities usually have arrangements for their guests to use a health club nearby. Find out exactly what you'll have access to (treadmills, stationary bikes, rowing machines, an indoor track or pool, aerobics classes) so you can be prepared to take advantage of it.
- When you pack, don't forget your walking or running shoes! Other items you might want to bring are a personal headset and your favorite music or audio walking tapes, exercise videotapes (if

program cautiously. Although you may be anxious to get started again, cut your program back by one-third if you've missed more than a week of exercise, and check with your doctor before resuming if you've been extremely sick. Don't be discouraged if you seem more out of shape than you want to be. The wisest thing is to build up to your previous fitness level carefully.

MAKING EXERCISE A PERMANENT PART OF YOUR LIFE

One Ph.D. candidate who wanted to do his thesis on the effects of *stopping* exercise had to abandon the project because he could find no volunteers! That's the kind of hold exercise can (and, we hope, *will*) get on you.

Make appointments with yourself to exercise, and keep them! Remind yourself frequently why you're doing this (for you!), and

the hotel has a compatible VCR), a jump rope (provided you have no knee problems and are familiar with this activity), and even—space allowing—a fold-up portable bicycle.

- Carry your exercise clothes, shoes, and equipment in a separate bag so you can get to them easily and at short notice. This can be very helpful if you take business trips with long airport layovers: Use the time between flights to walk up and down the airport concourse.
- If you're on a long driving trip, keep your exercise bag handy. Pull over at a park or rest stop, and spend 45 minutes to an hour walking or jogging—it will feel great after being confined to the car for hours.
- Include long walks or hikes in your vacation plans—it's a great way to get to museums, stores, or tourist attractions. Take fewer taxis and put more mileage on your walking shoes. In addition to the exercise benefits (and the money you'll save), you'll see a lot more of the city or countryside!

solicit support from your friends and family, just as you're doing for following the Lifetime Eating Plan. As you start to look better, you may run into some resistance, but don't let other people's envy get in the way. Just keep at it!

Give yourself "cues and prompts" to make sure you carry out your exercise plan: Lay your exercise clothes out the night before, so in the morning you can slip right into them and get going. Think of your walking, jogging, or aerobic workout at the health club or gym as an opportunity to socialize—to be with other people who are doing what *you're* doing to keep healthy. Consult your exercise planning chart as conscientiously as you consult your business calendar or "To Do" list—then keep those appointments with your own healthy destiny!

Take a moment to go over the points in this chapter, from seeing your doctor before you start out to choosing the right exercise(s) for you, and then set up your own weekly plan, using the following chart:

WEEKLY EXERCISE PLANNER

	Mon.	Tues.	Wed.	Thurs.	Fri.	Sat.	Sun.
Activity							
Hard or Easy							
Time							

RECORDING YOUR PROGRESS

Once you've decided what exercises you'll do, when you'll do them, and where, use a weekly exercise log like the one below to help you reach your goals. The ideal routine would be to alternate hard and easy days for six days of the week, with one day of rest (and do give yourself at least one day off). But if you opt for four or five days of

WEEKLY EXERCISE LOG

	Mon.	Tue.	Wed.	Thurs.	Fri.	Sat.	Sun.
Activity							
Hard or Easy							
Time							
THR							

exercise each week, make sure not to take two or more days off in a row, because it can be hard to get started again if you do. If you want a four-day program, try for a schedule such as Monday, Wednesday, Friday, and Saturday. Remember that consistency is the key to success.

CHAPTER 17

Success over Stress

The phone rings before you've had a chance to have breakfast. It's your boss, telling you to be in early this morning because an important meeting has been moved up. You look for the suit you were planning to wear and realize it's still at the cleaner's—and your only other decent one has a large stain on the jacket! As you search for a can of spot remover, your child stumbles into the bathroom. Sniffling and coughing, he announces he's "not feeling good." And he's not faking—you feel his forehead and know right away he's got a temperature. Suddenly you hear an ominous gurgling from the kitchen: The oatmeal is boiling over! As you rush out to rescue your breakfast, the phone rings again . . .

This is certainly a familiar scene from modern life, and there's no doubt that the demands and pressures of our lives sometimes threaten to virtually capsize us. Today, more people than ever before are working *and* running families, juggling more and more responsibilities, trying to deal with a noisier and more crowded world than we've ever known. Between traffic jams, endless lines at the supermarket, pressures on the job, and the assault of city noise, day and night, it's not at all surprising that so many people feel "too stressed," and that this complaint has become a currently popular, almost trendy, "disease."

WHAT IS STRESS?

These days, the term *stress* is so widely used—and misused—that it has developed several different meanings. One generally accepted definition, however, would be that stress is "the arousal of the mind and body in response to demands made on the individual." Now, that's not at all as complicated as it might sound. What it really means is simply that stress is our reaction to external events, but that it's internally driven. It means our thoughts and emotions are involved, as well as our physiological processes. And when we consider that everything we experience throughout the day calls for some kind of response on our part, it becomes clear that it means stress is always present to some degree in our lives. But that needn't be cause for concern: The key to dealing with stress is how we perceive the things that put demands on us, and how we react to them.

HOW ARE YOU DOING?

We each have our own personal stress barometer: Some people are happiest only when they're handling a lot of challenges, while others do better with less. It's all in what makes you feel best; in fact, too little can be as "wrong" as too much. Maybe you already know how you're doing in this department, and maybe you're satisfied with things the way they are. Or maybe you're not, and would like to get things into better balance. Either way, it's a good idea to step back and ask yourself a few questions.

How do you respond to the events in your life? How do you do from day to day, from moment to moment? Are you undermotivated? Feeling comfortably challenged? Or about to cave in? We naturally want to spend most of our time in the range where we feel "comfortably challenged." But because that range is different for everyone, what makes you feel just right may make someone else too stressed, or make another person feel bored.

And it's not always easy to maintain equilibrium in today's fast-paced world. Although some people actually feel that they're understimulated, the majority of people in our culture feel just the opposite. Why? Is life today simply filled with too many "stressful things"?

No, that's not it, as much as we might like to think so. First of all, remember that stress is *internally* driven. Strictly speaking, outside events—"things"—are not inherently "stressful." After all, they're just that—"things." Remember, too, that whether you feel over-stressed or not is just a matter of how you perceive, and react to, these outside events. Now if you're one of the many people who feel overstressed, you may be thinking, So what does *that* mean? That it's all *my* fault? Not at all. What we're really saying is that *you* have control—total control, in fact—over how stressed you feel.

Here's an example. Two people, each in their own car, are stuck in terrible rush-hour traffic. One quickly becomes frustrated with the delay and begins pounding on his horn and shouting at the cars ahead. The other person, realizing that the situation must just be waited out, uses the time to listen to the radio, or just organize her thoughts—and as soon as the traffic inches up to a corner phone booth, she hops out quickly to call the office and explain the delay. They're both in the same predicament, but each selects a different response. The first person clearly feels overstressed—not a product of the event itself, but, in fact, of his actual reaction to the event.

It's certainly easy to react the way the first person did; many of us do it automatically, and then end up feeling awful. The good news is that it doesn't have to be that way! When you think about it, we actually choose our reactions. So if you often feel "about to cave in" and are ready to make some changes, we hope these come as welcome words.

WHY BE CONCERNED?

You might be wondering what difference it makes, and why you can't just routinely blow off some steam. Quite frankly, it makes a lot of difference: Your health depends on it, in more ways than one. First of all, it's crucial to examine how you're feeling throughout the day, so you can have a realistic understanding of how you're reacting to what's going on in your life. For one thing, when you're feeling comfortably challenged it's easier to maintain the healthy eating and exercise habits you've worked so hard to establish. Few things will make you head for a martini and a big steak faster than a day during which you felt overstressed! But when things are in the right balance for you, you'll be able to face the crises head-on. Then you'll probably find yourself looking forward to an evening of exercise, a healthy dinner, and some pleasant time alone or with your family or friends.

The balanced life-style that's so critical for everyone—particularly in today's harried world—is one in which each of the elements complements and supports the others. For some people, there may be moments when striking and maintaining that balance seem like an impossibility. If you're one of them, reassure yourself: You *do* have options. And remember that a balanced life-style is one that will help you feel your best, because *every* facet of this life-style makes it easy to follow the Pritikin program every day.

And there's another, equally compelling reason why it's critical to maintain the balance that's right for you: The long-term effects of chronic stress can be *devastating* to your health. Prolonged or excess stress can attack your cardiovascular system, and can make you more susceptible to other illnesses as well. In short, too much stress can precipitate a whole host of physical dangers—which makes it far more crucial to be attuned to the signals your body gives you when it's under too much stress and to deal with things while they're still manageable.

Yet for a lot of different reasons, so many people don't. Paul T., a relatively young man with a wonderful family and a challenging job, found himself experiencing a variety of symptoms. Faced with mounting pressures at work, he rarely had the time—or the inclination—to have even a light lunch, so by the time he made it home at the end of the day he felt as though he'd been through the wringer, and frequently had a pounding headache as well. Several aspirin, a big dinner, and a strong drink became the evening norm, and although he was exhausted he often slept poorly. In the morning he'd take antacids for his upset stomach, groan at the fact that his clothes were getting tighter, and then start the demoralizing cycle all over again. It was only when he was struggling with the added burden of playing host to old friends who were visiting for two weeks that everything came to an abrupt halt: Paul suffered a serious heart attack at age thirty-eight. One of his first comments was, "I'm not surprised it happened—I just knew I couldn't go on the way I was. For a while I thought I could handle it all, but at some point I realized I was just pushing too hard."

Fortunately, Paul recovered and is now back on his chosen career track. But with the help of his family he's living a different kind of life—one that includes a good diet, a carefully monitored exercise program, and regular time out for himself. He's happy with his challenges, and he's in the right balance now for him. He learned a tough lesson, though—that we simply can't afford not to listen to what our bodies are telling us. The human body will withstand a lot of strain—but not without a protest! And not forever. Some signs and symptoms, left unattended, simply get worse, and our efforts to mask them (conscious or unconscious) are almost never successful in the long run.

STRESS SIGNALS

To appreciate the impact of stress overload in your own life, you have to become alert to its symptoms, which may be a little more difficult than you think. Many of us are so used to living with excess stress that we don't know any other way—and although we see and hear ourselves doing certain things, responding certain ways, we don't know how to interpret the messages we're getting. There's a good chance we've learned to respond in ways that just don't address the underlying problems.

There are literally dozens of different stress indicators. They can include frequent headaches; tension in the neck, shoulders, and/or back; attacks of arthritis or asthma; bowel irregularity; and digestive problems. A common stress indicator is disturbance in your sleep pattern. Then there's drinking, smoking, or eating to deal with tension, or resorting to tranquilizers or other chemical means of calming down. Other signals can range from impatience (things that didn't bother you before now set you off instantly) to sadness, anger, depression, boredom, "low-grade anxiety," fear, a lack of direction, a feeling that life has lost meaning, or a desire to be "rescued."

These signals are your body's way of alerting you, of letting you know something needs attention. Of course, they may be associated with a medical condition, or they may be indications of excess stress. One headache in three months may be nothing at all if you're otherwise doing fine and feeling "just right." But if headaches are an almost daily occurrence, and your stomach is sour most of the time, you owe it to yourself to acknowledge the symptoms, because ignoring them will rarely help chronic symptoms go away.

Take a closer look at these stress indicators, and think about the different signals. Do you have trouble sleeping? Do you have frequent muscle pain in your back or shoulders? Have you lost interest in any of the important aspects of your life? Are you often depressed—or angry? Once you've made yourself aware of the various signals, it will be easier to "hear" what your body is telling you the next time your day is interrupted by another throbbing headache.

So much of what we do is habit, so here's a good one to establish: Take a couple of moments each day to think about how you feel and how you're responding to what's going on. It's also very helpful, from time to time, to review your life-style in order to avoid overscheduling and to reset your priorities. Remember—*you're* in control! Knowing, and feeling, that you are will help with your responses to *all* of life's events, and will help keep your responses to the tough ones positive. In fact, research has shown that people who do respond positively to life's challenges can have a similarly positive influence on their health. These people are known as "hardy copers."

FINDING THE RIGHT APPROACH

Drs. Salvatore Maddi and Suzanne Kobasa compared the attitudes of these healthy "hardy copers" with those of people who actually fell ill from life's challenges. In studies of business executives and lawyers whose life-styles were all the same, Kobasa found one specific group of people who displayed behavioral characteristics that were associated with protection from physical illness. These people maintained a combination of three characteristics which together formed what the researchers termed the "stress-hardy" personality: *commitment, control,* and *challenge.*[1]

Commitment means a high degree of involvement in what you're doing, and it includes a desire to give it your best shot. Its opposite is alienation (as seen in children in orphanages who withdraw from everything around them). Commitment means working from a sense of purpose in yourself. In the business world, for example, this would mean being involved in, excited by, and delighted with your job—not just plugging away for a paycheck. Committed people care about the outcome of what they do; it means something to them. When faced with obstacles, you're more apt to solve problems than to become frustrated if you have a high level of commitment.

Control: People who feel a high degree of control in their lives aren't simply megalomaniacs who have to make sure things go their way—nor are they necessarily only the lucky folks who, because of money or independence, seem to be able to call their own shots. These people simply believe that, even in situations that may appear "uncontrollable," some action can be taken—and that taking action *can* make a difference, either in the particular situation they're in or in their life in general. Feeling you're "in control" means believing that you have more control than you might think and accepting responsibility (and credit!) for your decisions and actions. It means *choosing* not to be helpless, not to be a "victim" who blames the world for whatever happens to you.

Challenge is what you feel when you're faced with an obstacle you *want* to overcome: Challenged people believe that any situation, however difficult it may appear, is an opportunity to grow, improve, and *win.* When you see difficulty as challenge, you don't see only the negative, and you don't feel defeated by a situation you think you could never improve; you don't see changes as threats to your ego or a rigid status quo. The ability to find challenge in difficult situations is often associated with a sense of curiosity, and an intrigue with change. It cultivates flexibility and helps you to deal with the uncertainties of life. If you're strong in the "challenge" category, you'll be ready to bend with life—not resist it at all costs.

Remember, bad news or an abrupt change in plans doesn't have to mean the end of the world! For "hardy copers," these are the events that trigger opportunity, or perhaps the prospect of good, constructive change. These "possibility thinkers" focus on what they can do to make the situation better, even if it's not great to start with. (Sound a little too good to be true? Well, you don't have to be a Pollyanna to look at things this way. In fact, possibility thinkers are some of the most *realistic* people around. It's just that they've learned—sometimes, by the way, as a result of going through some very real changes—that there are almost always other options.)

The interaction of these three components—commitment, control, and challenge—helps produce the resilient personality that the Maddi/Kobasa study focused on, a style that contributes to "stress-hardiness." In fact, these attitudes even seem capable of protecting the *most* driven people—people who exhibit "Type A" behavior. Typical Type A's are impatient, feel an aggressive need to be right, to win, to do things more quickly and better than everyone else, and are driven to the point of irrationality. These people have long been associated with "coronary-prone patterns" and are assumed to be at greater risk of coronary heart disease.

But it's interesting to note that the Maddi/Kobasa study found that when Type A personalities *also* showed a high degree of commitment, control, and challenge, they exhibited *no stress/illness connection!* This, of course, is hardly a recommendation to follow Type A behavior—in point of fact, those ultra–Type A's who scored low on Kobasa's hardiness scale had the highest illness scores. (Researchers are now looking at Type A's in a new light, focusing on the idea that the hostility and anger aspects of Type A behavior may be the detrimental factors—not, perhaps, the long working hours and sense of time urgency. And hostility, of course, is *not* compatible with the stress-hardy traits of commitment, control, and challenge.)

"QUICK FIXES" DON'T WORK

Unfortunately, some people turn to "quick-fix" methods in an attempt to alleviate their excess stress, but fail to get at the underlying causes. It's easy to turn to what appears to be an instant remedy.

Many people hold on all day until "happy hour," when they can have a drink to "unwind." But alcohol has so much going against it that it simply can't be recommended as a stress reducer—or as any sort of panacea. High in calories and devoid of nutrients, it can only contribute to a weight problem (which itself can add stress), and consumed in excess it will impair judgment and eventually damage vital organs. Because alcohol is a nervous-system depressant that can leave you feeling anxious and depressed, using it to escape uncomfortable feelings is only a temporary ploy—it doesn't help you get to the root of what's bothering you. The effects of alcohol will wear off eventually, but the underlying issues will still be there.

Grabbing for a cigarette clearly isn't the answer, either—besides posing a terrible risk to cardiopulmonary health, smoking can actually *increase* tension rather than decrease it, since nicotine acts as a stimulant, and will get you more hyped up than you were in the first place. Tranquilizers and sleeping pills, on the other hand, act as depressants—and while they may seem to offer temporary relief, they can be addictive. Eating compulsively to calm down is also ineffective over the short *and* long runs: It's as temporary an escape as alcohol, and its long-term effect on your health can be devastating.

WHAT CAN WORK

There's no magic pill you can take to alleviate excess stress (and there probably never will be). But if you've decided it's time for a "rebalancing," it's good to know that there are several things you *can* do to stay comfortably challenged and productive at the same time. One of them is to be good to your body by following a healthy diet like the Pritikin Lifetime Eating Plan. It's really the perfect one— free of artificial stimulants and full of natural foods that don't tax your system.

And don't forget exercise! Exercise is one of the most wonderful, effective ways to combat tension buildup. Review its benefits, and you'll see why: Exercise lowers blood pressure and promotes the release of endorphins (natural opiates produced in the brain), giving you a natural "high" and a lasting sense of well-being. It makes you feel good about yourself, and thus more positive about facing life.

If you exercise alone, this gives you the chance to get off by yourself; if you work out with friends, exercising becomes a nice social break. Outdoor exercise provides a change of scene and the new perspective so vital to a positive point of view. We just can't say enough about the stress-reducing effects of exercise! They aren't only physical (considerable as the physical benefits are)—they promote a wonderful attitude. Attitude is, as you'll soon see, *crucial* to how you deal with life, and yet one more reason to make exercise a daily part of your life.

RELAXING AND RENEWING

Even the most stress-hardy need to take regular breaks. It's impossible to carry on successfully for weeks or even days on end without coming up for air—and foolish to think you can zoom along at a breakneck pace without paying a price at some point. What many people never seen to realize is that time out isn't only for repairing damage, it's for preventing it as well. Whatever you're doing, you'll do it better if your mind and body are in top form.

Most of us can't slip away whenever we'd like to for a rejuvenating weekend in a lavish resort—yet just about everyone who wants to can spare a few minutes from each day to nurture and renew themselves through some simple relaxation techniques. But how much relaxation, you might ask, can you possibly squeeze into just a few minutes? How much good can that little bit of time do?

You'd be surprised! For one thing, relaxation techniques can cleanse your mind of a lot of the mental clutter that makes it hard to think clearly and swiftly and to keep things in the proper perspective. And for another, they can actually help to lower your blood pressure—there's a sure stress-buster! With a clear mind and a calm body, you'll be in much better overall balance. You'll feel challenged rather than bombarded by life, and able to respond in the most positive fashion to whatever comes your way.

RELAXATION TECHNIQUES

At the mention of "relaxation techniques," especially if they have anything to do with meditation, some people automatically turn off—they think these techniques are silly, or are only for those seeking "spiritual" happiness. If you're one of those people (or if you've just never practiced meditation or relaxation exercises), don't worry: They're not necessary if you're following the Pritikin program, but they can be helpful. They're meant to relax you—and, in effect, "cleanse" you of tension.

From time to time, you can reexamine your life-style and commitments in order to see where you might make changes to reduce stress. If you'd like an on-the-spot remedy, relaxation techniques can be useful in those moments when you're especially stressed—when a deadline looms threateningly large, or when demands and crises at home or at work look as if they'll overturn you. And if you know you're under *chronic* stress (and therefore aren't following an optimal life-style), you owe it to yourself to practice these techniques on a regular basis: You don't want to suffer the debilitating effects of stress-induced illness or reach the point of complete exhaustion.

Relaxation techniques such as deep breathing, deep progressive relaxation, and mental focusing elicit what is known as the "relaxation response" in the human body—the exact opposite of the stress response. Heart rate goes down, blood pressure goes down, and the cellular need for oxygen is lessened. Respiration slows, stress hormones disappear from the bloodstream, and the brain produces alpha or theta waves, which indicate deep physiological and mental rest.[2] In fact, the relaxation response provides a deeper physiological rest than what you would derive from just lying down "relaxing," reading a book, or watching TV.

In one study in England, Dr. Chandra Patel tested two groups of people with high blood pressure: One group did the kind of deep relaxation you'll learn about in a moment, and the other group just reclined for a general relaxation. Blood pressure went down in both cases, but much more so in the deep-relaxation group. When the general-relaxation group was taught the deep-relaxation technique later, their blood pressures dropped to the same levels found in the deep-relaxation group.[3]

Being able to create the relaxation response anytime you want to is one way of staying in control of the stress in your life. When you give your body the rest it needs, you can go back to the "front lines" of your daily challenges with real physiological, and psychological, renewal. Think of these relaxation skills as your natural "martini replacement"—you just don't need addictive substances to relax!

QUIETING THE MIND

The constant chattering and background noise in your mind are some of the things that prevent you from being able to relax. But with a technique to help you quiet your mind, you can block out or at least quiet down all the little worries and thoughts that nag for your attention. You do this by giving yourself only *one thing* to focus on.

Herbert Benson, a distinguished Harvard physician who has extensively documented the benefits of mental concentration practices, offers research that shows that the relaxation response helps in a number of ways. At Benson's Mind/Body Clinic at Harvard, participants are taught to use mental focusing or concentration techniques twice a day for 10 to 20 minutes in order to improve their ability to handle the stress-related component of conditions such as cardiovascular disease, hypertension, cancer, AIDS, and infertility. Benson and his associates have shown that these techniques also allow for a balancing of the brain waves in the right and left hemispheres of the brain[4] (a balancing that may be related to improvement in learning—this is under investigation by scientists now).

Getting the most you can from a relaxation-response exercise requires motivation and practice—and although you'll feel some immediate positive effects, you'll need to do the exercise regularly to get the full benefit. But this is a simple technique, one that is easy to learn and do, and we've set it out in the box on the following page.

Keep the following things in mind about this effective relaxation technique: First, try to maintain a passive attitude—that is, don't judge your performance. When your mind wanders from your focus word, as it inevitably will, gently bring it back. But don't scold yourself—everyone experiences some mind-wandering. Just bring yourself back gently each time, returning your attention again to the focus word, and gradually your mind will begin to quiet down. Once you're able to sustain your concentration upon the focus word, you'll experience the deep quieting of the mind that elicits the relaxation response in the body. This is a marvelously refreshing exercise—more refreshing the more you practice it. Some people like to do this for 10 minutes in the morning before going to work; in the evening

MENTAL CONCENTRATION EXERCISE

Let's begin by selecting a "focus" word to concentrate on. It can be any simple word that you like, and can be something out of your unique experience or background. Some people choose a word like "love," "truth," "peace," or "life," a color or a number, or just "let go" or "calm." The object of the exercise is to quiet your mind by keeping your focus word at the forefront of your attention.

Once you have your focus word, you're ready to begin.

1. Sit up straight, but not stiff. Keep your shoulders back and your spine in alignment (if you slump you'll have a tendency to fall asleep). Uncross your arms and legs. You can keep your hands in any comfortable position in your lap. Close your eyes—this makes it easier to concentrate.
2. Now go over your body from head to toes, mentally relaxing and releasing any tension you find. Let your shoulders drop and relax (but still don't slump).
3. Next, observe your natural breathing process for just a few moments. There's no need to control it—just be aware of your breath coming and going gently.
4. Now, in the same way you just observed your breathing without trying to control it, place your focus word at the forefront of your attention. Keep your eyes closed, keep the word before you, and focus on it. If your mind wanders, just bring it gently back to the focus word. If you like, you can say the word quietly to yourself as you exhale, since the rhythm of your breathing may help you focus more easily on your word. Or just use the word alone. Repeat it at your regular rate of speaking, or with the timing of each exhalation—whatever you prefer. Continue for at least 5 minutes.

before bed is also a good time—whatever fits your schedule. Once this focusing technique becomes a part of your daily routine, you won't want to miss a session. Give yourself some time to make the relaxation response a regular part of your life—the benefits are greater than you imagine.

There are many other types of relaxation techniques—more than one book could possibly teach you. Once you awaken your interest in summoning the relaxation response (which we hope will happen as a result of practicing the exercise you've just learned), you may want to explore *progressive relaxation,* which involves concentrating on a series of body parts, tightening muscle groups, becoming conscious of how tension feels, and then releasing tension; *meditation techniques; deep breathing;* and *positive imagery.* There is virtually a wealth of ways you can quiet your mind, and nurture yourself to real rejuvenation.

ENJOY LIFE!

Remember—*you're* in control! And you do have options. It may not come overnight, but once you start to see challenging situations as inevitable but surmountable—as opportunities to grow rather than reasons to panic, lash out, or flee—you will do more for your health than may at first be apparent. What you'll be doing for yourself, across the board, sounds deceptively simple, perhaps even unimportant: You'll be making yourself more *comfortable* with the world around you. However, that feeling of greater ease—the sense that you've got more control over your feelings, your environment, and the unpredictable events in your life—is an immeasurable asset, one that not only protects you from a number of life-threatening illnesses, but also makes it possible for you to maintain a balanced life-style and *enjoy* life more. The desire to enjoy life (and for as long as possible) is, after all, a large motivation for taking care of yourself, isn't it? It just doesn't make sense not to ease your path in every way you can. Staying attuned to yourself, and learning to react positively to life's events, will go a long way toward doing just that.

So will the "positive-approach" guidelines you'll learn about next!

CHAPTER 18

Making the Pritikin Program Permanent by Keeping It S.I.M.P.L.E.

Now that you're ready to make some very important—and very positive!—changes in your life, it's natural to wonder how you make the Pritikin program's practical guidelines *stick*. Are there ways to make the transition from an unhealthy life-style to a healthy one that won't make you feel as if you're doomed to failure—that it's all too much? Naturally, you may have some big changes ahead of you. And change, as you now know, can bring its share of stress. But now you know how to deal with that stress, how to keep yourself from feeling overwhelmed and build a positive attitude—you realize that you *do* have the power to reach your good health goals, step by step.

To get you started, we've drawn on our own experience, and the experience of thousands of Pritikin program participants, to devise an approach that seems to work for just about everyone who wants to make the Pritikin program an ongoing part of their life.

If there's a theme to all of this, it's one you've heard from us already: "Progress, not perfection." Everyone who follows the Pritikin program successfully for a long period of time aims for—and acknowledges—progress, because perfection is difficult, if not impossible, to attain. It's far better to congratulate yourself for taking the *next* step to good health than it is to berate yourself for not having reached your final goal right away (which, when you think

336

about it, is impossible!). The exciting journey you've already undertaken toward new energy, greater health, and a strong sense of well-being will continue at exactly the pace you started at: step by step. We've said before that if an eating or exercise program isn't enjoyable, you probably won't keep at it for long. That principle of enjoyment and "livability" is the one we bring to our whole Pritikin program—and it's the principle behind what we've appropriately named the "S.I.M.P.L.E." approach. Here's what the letters mean:

S = Self-motivate by keeping your goals in mind
I = Identify common eating triggers
M = Make new choices
P = Plan ahead
L = Learn to reward your positive efforts
E = Engineer your environment for success

"But I thought you said this was going to be *simple!*" you say. "Now it sounds as if you're telling me to change everything in my life!"

Yes, we *are* asking you to take a new look at what you're doing to yourself—nutritionally, physically, and emotionally. But every one of our "S.I.M.P.L.E." suggestions is designed to help you do just that, and to help you along your way to renewed health. Let's go through the list so you can see for yourself.

S = SELF-MOTIVATE

Here's where we repeat "Focus on your goals." (This does *not* mean "Berate yourself because you haven't attained your goals yet.") We've found that it's easiest to institute successful, healthy changes when you simply remind yourself why you're doing it!

Imagine that you're grocery shopping, walking down the frozen-food aisle past stacks and stacks of ice cream cartons in every imaginable flavor. Then you move into the dairy aisle and see all that low-fat yogurt (filled with sugary preserves), and finally, at the very end of the row, you see the cartons of plain nonfat yogurt. But look at all that wonderful sweet stuff!

Stop. This is where we'd like you to take a deep breath and remember what all the fat and sugar you're passing up will do to you if you *do* indulge. This is the time to make an active, conscious choice—a choice, by the way, that does not have to limit you to plain nonfat yogurt: A tablespoon of Pritikin brand fruit spread or some fresh berries or half a sliced banana will transform your no-fat fare into something every bit as good as the fatty alternatives you've passed by. Give yourself a little pinch around the middle. Remind yourself of what your doctor said at your last visit. That's what "self-motivate" means.

The next time you feel tempted by those chocolate-chip cookies that are just crying out for your attention, take a moment to review the reasons you want to change your diet: to lose weight, lower your cholesterol, reduce hypertension, feel more energetic, look years younger. Remember: You're doing all this for *yourself*. You're giving yourself a continuing gift no one else can make possible—the gift of good health.

I = IDENTIFY COMMON EATING TRIGGERS

It's no secret that food does more than taste good and fill our stomachs. Food is comfort. Solace. A reward. It may be what you reach for when you're bored, tense, happy, depressed, reading, watching television, listening to the stereo, talking on the phone, worrying about a project at work. What you may not quite have grasped, however, is that each of these situations acts as a "trigger"—a catalyst or stimulus that in this case provokes hand-to-mouth action. Everything around us can turn into a cue to eat: We're so used to grabbing food to calm down, to lessen the impact of even minor upsets or stresses. You may not *think* you're following cues when you reach for the potato chips, but if you keep a short log of what you eat and when—along with what you're doing or feeling when you eat—you'll be astonished at how regular your patterns are.

From infancy on, food comes to mean "love" or "reward": As we grew up, weren't we given ice cream for having been good? Cake for dessert because we managed to get through our lima beans? It's no wonder that, as adults, we're virtually addicted to fatty, sugary sweets, which have come to represent even more than something that "tastes good." We still feel the need to reward or placate ourselves, and hence our love affair with quick-fix junk food.

We'd like you to reward yourself, too—but with something that will really *be* a reward! Once you've identified the triggers that are associated with reaching for unhealthy food, use that energy to reach for a handful of grapes, a juicy orange, a slice of whole-grain bread, or a stick of fresh celery. This leads us to our next suggestion.

M = MAKE NEW CHOICES

This may be the most exhilarating revelation of all: the fact that we have a *choice*. That when we feel the cue to eat something we know is unhealthy, we can stop for a moment, focus on what it is that's provoking us to eat, and, as clearly as we can, figure out what our real options are. *That's* what freedom of choice means. Your first disappointed response might be that you don't feel "free" anymore to eat french fries, fatty meats, butter, and ice cream. But when you take a moment to remind yourself what these foods are going to do to you if you eat them (clog your arteries, increase your cholesterol and blood pressure, thicken your middle, and, quite frankly, dramatically increase your chances of developing life-threatening disease)—and what the healthy foods will do for you if you eat *them* (lower your serum cholesterol, help you lose excess body fat, improve your cardiovascular health)—you're truly using your free will and your intellect to choose a better, healthier alternative.

And the alternative doesn't always have to be another kind of food. What about doing some stretching or aerobic exercise? Lydia B., a free-lance writer, came up with an ingenious solution that made new use of her cookie jar. It was once filled to the brim with chocolate-chip cookies, to which she turned whenever she felt the least twinge of writer's block or anxiety about her mother, the rent, the weather, an upcoming date, or the cat getting fur on the couch. Now when she feels anxiety, she still reaches into the cookie jar—but she takes out one of several notes to herself that say things like "Go for a walk," "Play with the cat," "Water the plants," "Take a bike ride," "Call a friend." She may also, however, have a slice of Apple-Date Cake! (Remember, eat if you are hungry—but eat the right things.)

Alternatives abound. Take the time to consider your choices when you're planning your menu, making up your shopping list, or selecting food from the grocery shelves. *You* are always in control, no matter how strongly the wrong foods seem to plead with you to take them home. That moment when you pull back on the reins, take a breath, and really *see* what you're about to do—that moment of "time out"—is crucial. And when you feel as if you just might cave in, remember that you've *always* got the power to stop, take a step back, and assess the situation more clearly. Sometimes a craving for food really does mean you're hungry—so eat! But have frozen non-fat yogurt or fresh fruit sorbet instead of ice cream.

The trick to controlling your behavior is recognizing that the *small* steps, the seemingly insignificant changes (like popping a grape into your mouth instead of a peanut), do add up. Take a moment to concentrate on the immediate actions you *do* have the power to take—not on the ultimate goals that can be attained only with time.

Say you want to lose 25 pounds, but you feel exasperated because you can't change everything *right now*. Our immediate-gratification "buttons" always seem to demand pushing. But when you rail at the frustration of having to lose that weight slowly, you can take "time out" and remind yourself it *is* coming off—that you're doing exactly what you need to do to take (and keep) it off. The three or four months it takes to lose the weight are nothing compared to the *years* ahead of enjoying life at your proper weight—you'll barely remember a few months of "waiting" during which that weight loss seemed impossible!

P = PLAN AHEAD

You're exhausted and hungry after a long day and suddenly realize there's nothing in the kitchen—so you rush out to get to the supermarket before it closes. Once there, you're overwhelmed by the rows and rows of colorful, tempting foods—potato chips, ice cream, ready-to-eat fried chicken, every food you know is "bad" for you. And the only things you can think of that are *healthy* seem as if they would take forever to make. You're hungry and confused, and you just can't think of much that is good for you. If only you'd made a shopping list!

Sometimes the simplest preparation tactics can avert disaster: You're certainly never more vulnerable than when you're wandering around the supermarket hungry! In this case, as in most others as well, the most obvious preventive measure is the best: Make up a shopping list, and then *stick to what's on it.* You'll develop the strength to say no to the unhealthy stuff if you make your list an ironclad guide. *If it's not on it, don't buy it!*

This will help you with our next suggestion: Don't keep foods you don't want to eat in the house. Again, it sounds too obvious to bear stating, but if you don't keep unhealthy foods, you won't eat them. Plan ahead by ridding your shelves of these foods now, so they're not there to tempt you. (And remember our "S" suggestion—self-motivation—as you discard the food you know just isn't healthy for you: Remind yourself why you're doing all this!)

Another way to plan ahead is to remember our exercise advice, as well as our relaxation advice, and then schedule time for both in your day. It's *your* choice: Loll around in front of the television, or take an invigorating walk. Fall into bed and lie awake with a lot on your mind, or spend 10 minutes quieting your mind with the help of our relaxation-response technique. You'll truly be set up for success when you're prepared, ahead of time, with these antidotes to tension and anxiety.

L = LEARN TO REWARD YOUR POSITIVE EFFORTS

When you first start to make new choices—just like a baby who makes his first "choice" to try to walk—they won't seem automatic. At the beginning, you'll be aware of some effort; after all, you're embarking on a program to change habits you've probably had for a lifetime. Naturally you'll resist some of these changes. So what can you do when you've really accomplished something? Reward yourself!

Don't wait until you're the perfect you, until you've achieved the ultimate goal of a 25-pound weight loss or a drop of 50 mg/dl in your cholesterol—celebrate every small step you take in the right direction. Make these little celebrations personal and specific, something that really will seem like a reward: a massage, a facial, an afternoon at the movies, a visit to a museum, tickets to a ball game or the theater.

E = ENGINEER YOUR ENVIRONMENT

Like Alice in the strange world of Wonderland, sometimes we feel totally at the mercy of our environment. Either the fast-food lunches our coworkers carry past our desks, or the attitudes of the people in our lives—loved ones, friends, and acquaintances, people who say, "Oh, come on—you can have just *one* . . ." or "You're not really *fat* . . ." or "Are you trying to prove you're a saint?" It's tough to face the hurt look in your sister's eyes when you turn down her liver pâté or not be offended yourself by the envy-inspired taunts of unsupportive "friends" who say, "You don't look like you've lost *that* much weight!" Sometimes the world can seem like a mine field when you're attempting to make healthy changes in what you eat—full of temptations and unhelpful comments, all seemingly geared to put you off track.

Being aware of what's working for or against you is the first step in learning to engineer your environment so that you've got the best chance of success. Here are some more tips:

- Take a good look at your family role models: Did anyone—or does anyone now—rely on eating (particularly junk food) to combat emotions? What excuses do other members of your family make when they eat the wrong foods, if they do? How much value do they place on health and fitness? Will they support you in your efforts to lose weight and/or reduce disease risk factors?
- Communicate as openly and actively as you can with your family and friends: Tell them what you want and be specific about how you'd like them to support you. You may even find that one or more of the people closest to you will want to join in! It can be a tremendous boon to stick to a good healthy plan with another person: Support is crucial. To get your kids to support you, let them know how good you feel about what you're doing. It's never too early to start sending the message that our health depends on what we do to, and for, ourselves.
- There's another side to the coin, of course: Don't turn into a pushy evangelist. This may be harder to do than you can foresee. The benefits of the Pritikin plan are so wonderful that you'll *want* to go around

telling people what they're doing wrong, or how what they're eating is affecting their health. The problem is, they'll turn off—just as you would if someone tried to force it on you, however well intentioned. Just be your own best example; simply do what you know is right for yourself, and your actions will be more persuasive than a lecture could possibly be. You want to cultivate support—not resentment—in the people around you. And it helps to get as much support, especially at the beginning, as you can!

• Identify the nonsupportive people, or "saboteurs," in your midst, the ones who will try to undermine your efforts. Consciously or not—and for a variety of reasons ranging from envy to their inability to cope with change—even your closest loved ones may try to thwart you by bringing home candy or coaxing you to have second helpings of fish, meat, or poultry. Seek out, to the degree you can, those people whose values and goals most closely match your own. Once the ones who really care about you get the message that you're serious, you may be surprised at the result. One woman whose office birthday party was traditionally celebrated with an elaborate butter-cream cake was treated by her co-workers to an equally delicious healthy cake when it became clear that she really wanted to stick to the Pritikin plan. (The cake was so good, some of her colleagues are now trying the Pritikin plan themselves!)

• As we've suggested before, keep problem foods out of sight—or, better still, out of your kitchen and home entirely!

• Bring fresh fruit, whole-grain bread, or raw vegetables to work, to enjoy at coffee break. And keep a supply of herb tea bags to use instead of coffee. If there's an office party, offer to bring in some Tortilla Chips and Artichoke Pâté to replace the predictable high-fat canapés—then, even if everyone else is wrapped up in their pigs-in-blankets, at least you'll have something to eat! (They'll be delighted, too, when they discover how good the food you've brought in is.)

• When you're feeling stressed out and you've got a few minutes, take off and do a little stretching or a simple relaxation exercise (refer again to Chapters 16 and 17 for ideas): It's guaranteed to relax you when you need it.

• Keep a comfortable pair of walking shoes at your desk so you can take a brisk walk during lunch hour; use the stairs instead of the elevator, if it's feasible. You can build in a little extra activity in a lot of different ways that will occur to you throughout your day.

• Investigate the possibility of installing a small refrigerator and/or microwave oven at work—perhaps your colleagues will want to go in on it with you. One lucky department at a major ad agency was blessed by an enlightened boss who supplied his staff with frozen Pritikin Quick

Cuisine™ meals—which were microwaved for lunch. Even if you're not equally lucky, you just might be able to turn your workplace into as "safe" an eating place as your own home is—and avoid the temptations of the local coffee shop.

There are so many other ways to set yourself up for success (in fact, as you progress on the Pritikin program, you'll probably come up with a few pointers for *us*). You'll find yourself thinking of them spontaneously—like cultivating friends who are as committed to staying slim and healthy as you are. Being around people who've mastered what you'd like to learn is one of the best ways of learning it yourself. And soon *you'll* be the powerful example to others, who'll see how complete a transformation they, too, can experience.

In fact, one of the very best things about the Pritikin program is that it's just that—complete. It addresses all the major risk factors in a beautifully comprehensive way, because it encompasses not just what you eat, but how you live. It's a way of life.

Positive, visible results tell our story best. Soon it will be your story, too—we're sure of it. A story of glowing good health, renewed energy, and vigor—for a lifetime!

For information about Pritikin brand food products, write to:

Pritikin Systems, Inc.
P.O. Box 9003
Chicago, IL 60604-9003

For information about the Pritikin program, write to:

Pritikin Systems, Inc.
Box 573
1223 Wilshire Blvd.
Santa Monica, CA 90403

Acknowledgments

I would like to express my gratitude to the people who were of invaluable assistance in the writing of this book.

I am grateful to the staff at the Pritikin Longevity Center who were so helpful in the creation of this book, including Ellen Bauersfeld, M.S., R.D., Lisa Nicholson, M.S., R.D., Susan Massaron, Director of the Pritikin Longevity Center Cooking School, and Hortensia Calderon for their special help in developing menus and recipes; Alison Buckley, Robbie Gluckson, Eugenia Killoran, and David Liff of the Marketing Department for their creative contributions; Jennifer Owen for her assistance in preparing the manuscript; Claire Trazenfeld for her assistance and editorial advice; Diane Hanson, Ph.D., R.N., for managing this large project from start to finish; and Lorraine Kubernach for her editing talents and her skill in coordinating the parts and people involved.

Thanks to all the Pritikin Systems, Inc., staff who so generously gave of their time to review the manuscript and offer valuable suggestions.

I am especially indebted to all the alumni of the Pritikin Centers who have participated in our programs. I have learned a great deal from their experiences.

Thanks are also due to Guy Kettelhack, whose editorial and writing skills helped make this book come together. His innovative handling of this material made his contribution vital.

Thanks also go to Barbara Becker. Her patience and attention to detail, along with her talents for writing and editing, all added immeasurably to this book.

And special thanks to my mother, Ilene Pritikin.

346

Notes

INTRODUCTION

1. Hans Diehl and Don Mannerberg. "Hypertension, hyperlipidaemia, angina and coronary heart disease," in H. C. Trowell and D. P. Burkitt, eds., *Western Diseases: Their Emergence and Prevention.* Cambridge, MA: Harvard University Press, 1981.
2. R. James Barnard et al. "Effects of an intensive exercise and nutrition program on patients with coronary artery disease: Five-year follow-up." *Journal of Cardiac Rehabilitation,* 3:183–190, 1983.
3. Dean M. Ornish et al. "Can lifestyle changes reverse atherosclerosis?" *Circulation,* supplement (abstracts from the 61st Scientific Sessions, American Heart Association), 14:11, 1988.

CHAPTER 1

1. "Dietary guidelines for healthy American adults. A statement for physicians and health professionals by the Nutrition Committee, American Heart Association." *Circulation,* 77:721A–724A, 1988.
2. *The Surgeon General's Report on Nutrition.* U.S. Department of Health and Human Services, 1988.
3. Dean M. Ornish et al. "Can lifestyle changes reverse atherosclerosis?" *Circulation,* supplement (abstracts from the 61st Scientific Sessions, American Heart Association), 14:11, 1988.

CHAPTER 2

1. James J. Kenney, R. James Barnard, and John Hall. "Nutritional adequacy with long-term use of the Pritikin diet." Unpublished data presented at the 71st American Dietetic Association meeting, October 1988.

CHAPTER 3

1. R. R. Kohn. *Principles of Mammalian Aging,* 2nd edition. Englewood Cliffs, NJ: Prentice-Hall, 1978.
2. C. M. McCay et al. "Retarded growth, life span, ultimate body size and age changes in the albino rat after feeding diets restricted in calories." *Journal of Nutrition,* 18:1–13, 1939.
3. Lauren Lissner et al. "Dietary fat and the regulation of energy intake in human subjects." *American Journal of Clinical Nutrition,* 46:886–892, 1987.
4. Sheldon Saul Hendler. *The Complete Guide to Anti-Aging Nutrients.* New York: Simon and Schuster, 1984.

CHAPTER 4

1. Hans Diehl and Don Mannerberg. "Hypertension, hyperlipidaemia, angina and coronary heart disease," in H. C. Trowell and D. P. Burkitt, eds., *Western Diseases: Their Emergence and Prevention.* Cambridge, MA: Harvard University Press, 1981.
2. Stephen Inkeles and Daniel Eisenberg. "Hyperlipidemia and coronary atherosclerosis: A review." *Medicine,* 60:110–123, 1981.
3. S. L. Connor et al. "The cholesterol/saturated fat index: An indication of the hypercholesterolemic and atherogenic potential of food." *Lancet,* 1:1229–1232, 1986.
4. National Research Council. *Diet and Health: Implications for Reducing Chronic Disease Risk.* Washington, DC: National Academy Press, 1989.
5. American Heart Association. "Joint statement of the Nutrition Committee and the Council of Arteriosclerosis: Recommendations for the treatment of hyperlipidemia in adults." *Circulation,* 69:1065A–1090A, 1984.
6. W. S. Harris et al. "Effects of a low-saturated-fat, low-cholesterol fish oil supplement in hypertriglyceride patients." *Annals of Internal Medicine,* 109:465–470, 1988.

7. D. M. Demke et al. "Effects of a fish oil concentrate on patients with hypercholesterolemia." *Atherosclerosis,* 70:73–80, 1988.

8. L. V. Lefferts. "Good fish, bad fish." *Nutrition Action Health Letter,* 15:5–7, 1988.

9. H. Glauber et al. "Adverse metabolic effect of omega-3 fatty acids in non-insulin-dependent diabetes mellitus." *American Internal Medicine,* 108:663–668, 1988.

10. Scott Grundy et al. "Comparison of monounsaturated fatty acids and carbohydrates for reducing raised levels of plasma cholesterol in man." *American Journal of Clinical Nutrition,* 47:965–969, 1988.

11. National Research Council, *Diet and Health.*

CHAPTER 5

1. J. Stamler, D. Wentworth, and J. D. Neaton. "Is the relationship between serum cholesterol and risk of premature death from coronary heart disease continuous or graded? Finding in 356,222 primary screenees of the Multiple Risk Factor Intervention Trial (MRFIT)." *Journal of the American Medical Association,* 256:2873–2878, 1986.

2. "Expert panel: Report of the National Cholesterol Education Program Expert Panel on Detection, Evaluation and Treatment of High Blood Cholesterol in Adults." *Archives of Internal Medicine,* 148:36–69, 1988.

3. William P. Castelli. "The cholesterol beat . . . All angles on the story." *Heart Corps,* 1(5):16–17, 1989.

4. Stephen Inkeles and David Eisenberg. "Hyperlipidemia and coronary atherosclerosis: A review." *Medicine,* 60:110–123, 1981.

5. N. M. Kaplan and J. Stamler. *Prevention of Coronary Heart Disease: Practical Management of Risk Factors.* Philadelphia: W. B. Saunders, 1983.

6. Stamler et al., "Relationship between serum cholesterol," *Journal of the American Medical Association.*

7. W. F. Enos et al. "Pathogenesis of coronary disease in American soldiers killed in Korea." *Journal of the American Medical Association,* 158:192, 1955.

8. J. J. McNamara et al. "Coronary artery disease in combat casualties in Vietnam." *Journal of the American Medical Association,* 216:1185, 1971.

9. "Expert panel," *Archives of Internal Medicine.*

10. D. H. Blankenhorn et al. "Beneficial effects of combined colestipol-niacin therapy on coronary atherosclerosis and coronary venous bypass grafts." *Journal of the American Medical Association,* 257:3233–3240, 1987.

11. Lipid Research Clinic's Program. "The Lipid Research Clinic's coro-

nary primary prevention trial results." *Journal of the American Medical Association,* 251:351–371, 1984.

12. Inkeles and Eisenberg, "Hyperlipidemia," *Medicine.*

13. Castelli, "Cholesterol beat," *Heart Corps.*

14. Dean M. Ornish et al. "Can lifestyle changes reverse atherosclerosis?" *Circulation,* supplement (abstracts from the 61st Scientific Sessions, American Heart Association), 14:11, 1988.

15. Ancel Keys et al. "HDL serum cholesterol and 21-year mortality of men in Finland." *International Journal of Epidemiology,* 13:428–435, 1984.

16. W. E. Connor et al. "The plasma lipids, lipoproteins and diet of the Tarahumara Indians of Mexico." *American Journal of Clinical Nutrition,* 31:1131, 1978.

17. Keys et al., "HDL serum cholesterol," *International Journal of Epidemiology.*

18. "Expert panel," *Archives of Internal Medicine.*

19. J. Stamler and R. Shekelle. "Dietary cholesterol and human coronary heart disease: The epidemiologic evidence." *Archives of Pathological Laboratory Medicine,* 112:1032–1040, 1988.

20. D. B. Zilversmit. "Atherogenesis: A postprandial phenomenon." *Circulation,* 60:473, 1979.

21. Stamler and Shekelle, "Dietary Cholesterol," *Archives of Pathological Laboratory Medicine.*

22. R. James Barnard et al. "Effects of an intensive, short-term exercise and nutrition program on patients with ischemic heart disease." *Journal of Cardiac Rehabilitation,* 1:99–105, 1981.

23. M. B. Rosenthal et al. "Effects of a high-complex-carbohydrate, low-fat, low-cholesterol diet on serum lipids and estradiol." *American Journal of Medicine,* 78:23–27, 1985.

24. Hans Diehl and Don Mannerberg. "Hypertension, hyperlipidaemia, angina and coronary heart disease," in H. C. Trowell and D. P. Burkitt, eds., *Western Diseases: Their Emergence and Prevention.* Cambridge, MA: Harvard University Press, 1981.

25. Lipid Research, "Coronary primary prevention," *Journal of the American Medical Association.*

26. D. Kromhaut and C. de L. Coulander. "Diet, prevalence and 10-year mortality from coronary heart disease in 871 middle-aged men: The Zutphen study." *American Journal of Epidemiology,* 119:733–741, 1984.

CHAPTER 6

1. National Research Council. *Diet and Health: Implications for Reducing Chronic Disease Risk.* Washington, DC: National Academy Press, 1989.

2. Ibid.
3. J. Tuomilehto et al. "Nutrition-related determinants of blood pressure." *Preventive Medicine*, 14:413–427, 1985.
4. Theodore Kurtz et al. "Salt-sensitive essential hypertension in men: Is the sodium ion alone important?" *New England Journal of Medicine*, 317:1043–1048, 1987.
5. Tuomilehto et al., "Nutrition-related determinants," *Preventive Medicine*.
6. R. James Barnard et al. "Effects of a high-complex-carbohydrate diet and daily walking on blood pressure and medication status of hypertensive patients." *Journal of Cardiac Rehabilitation*, 3:389–846, 1983.
7. Tuomilehto et al., "Nutrition-related determinants," *Preventive Medicine*.
8. O. Ophir et al. "Low blood pressure in vegetarians: The possible role of potassium." *American Journal of Clinical Nutrition*, 37:755–762, 1983.
9. Eaton S. Boyd and Melvin Konner. "Paleolithic nutrition: A consideration of its nature and current implications." *New England Journal of Medicine*, 312:283–289, 1985.

CHAPTER 7

1. Walter Kempner. "Treatment of heart and kidney disease and of hypertensive and arteriosclerotic vascular disease with the rice diet." *Annals of Internal Medicine*, 31:821–856, 1949.
2. C. J. Lee et al. "Nitrogen retention of young men fed rice with or without supplementary chicken." *American Journal of Clinical Nutrition*, 24:318–323, 1971.
3. Ibid.
4. E. Kofranyi and F. Jekat. "The determination of the biological value of dietary protein. XI. The effect of methionine on nitrogen requirement." *Annals of Physiological Chemistry*, 342:248, 1965.
5. J. Knapp et al. "Growth and nitrogen balance in infants fed cereal proteins." *American Journal of Clinical Nutrition*, 26:586–590, 1973.
6. S. Bolomchi et al. "Wheat flour as a source of protein for adult human subjects." *American Journal of Clinical Nutrition*, 21:827–835, 1968.
7. William A. Forsythe et al. "Dietary protein effects on cholesterol and lipoprotein concentration: A review." *Journal of the American College of Nutrition*, 5:533–547, 1986.
8. National Research Council. *Report of the Committee on Diet, Nutrition and Cancer.* (Food and Nutrition Board, Assembly of Life Sciences.) Washington, DC: National Academy Press, 1982.

9. L. Solomon. "Osteoporosis and fracture of the femoral neck in the South African Bantu." *Journal of Bone and Joint Surgery*, 50B:2, 1968.

10. H. M. Linkswiler et al. "Calcium retention of young adult males as affected by level of protein and of calcium intake." *Transactions of the New York Academy of Sciences*, Series II, 36:333–340, 1974.

11. L. Allen. "Protein-induced hypercalciuria: A longer-term study." *American Journal of Clinical Nutrition*, 32:741, 1979.

12. S. Schuette. "Studies on the mechanism of protein-induced hypercalciuria in older men and women." *Journal of Nutrition*, 110:305, 1980.

13. M. Hegsted. "Urinary calcium and calcium balance in young men as affected by level of protein and phosphorus intake." *Journal of Nutrition*, 111:553, 1981.

14. G. D. Talbott and R. Frayser. "Hyperlipidaemia: A cause of decreased oxygen saturation." *Nature*, 200:684, 1963.

CHAPTER 8

1. U.S. Department of Health and Human Services, Public Health Service, National Institutes of Health. *National Cancer Institute Monograph: Cancer Control Objectives for the Nation: 1985–2000* (NIH Publication #86–2880). Washington, DC: United States Government Printing Office, 1986.

2. D. P. Burkitt and H. C. Trowell. *Refined Carbohydrate Foods and Disease: Some Implications of Dietary Fiber*. London: Academic Press, 1975.

3. J. W. Anderson et al. "Hypocholesterolemic effects of oat-bran or bean intake for hypercholesterolemic men." *American Journal of Clinical Nutrition*, 40:1146–1155, 1984.

4. J. W. Anderson et al. "Dietary fiber and diabetes: A comprehensive review and practical application." *Journal of the American Dietetic Association*, 87:1189–1197, 1987.

5. J. Stevens et al. "Effect of psyllium gum and wheat bran on spontaneous energy intake." *American Journal of Clinical Nutrition*, 46:812–817, 1987.

6. A. R. P. Walker et al. "Studies in human mineral metabolism. I. The effect of bread rich in phytate phosphorus on the metabolism of certain mineral salts with special reference to calcium." *Biochemical Journal*, 42:452–462, 1948.

7. E. R. Morris et al. "Trace element nutritive response of adult men consuming dephytinized or nondephytinized wheat bran," in D. D. Hemphill, *Trace Substances in Environmental Health XIV*. Columbia, MO: University of Missouri Press, 1980.

8. J. W. Anderson et al. "Mineral and vitamin status on high fiber diets: Long-term studies of diabetic patients." *Diabetes Care,* 3:38–40, 1980.
9. James J. Kenney, R. James Barnard, and John Hall. "Nutritional adequacy with long-term use of the Pritikin diet." Unpublished data presented at the 71st American Dietetic Association meeting, October 1988.
10. American Institute for Cancer Research. *Dietary Fiber to Lower Cancer Risk.* Washington, DC: American Institute for Cancer Research, 1988.

CHAPTER 9

1. Donald S. Miller et al. "Experimental study of overeating low- or high-protein diets." *American Journal of Clinical Nutrition,* 20:1212–1222, 1967.
2. K. Donato and D. M. Hegsted. "Efficiency of utilization of various sources of energy for growth." Proceedings, National Academy of Science (USA) 82:4866–4870, 1985.
3. H. C. Trowell and D. P. Burkitt, eds. *Western Diseases: Their Emergence and Prevention.* Cambridge, MA: Harvard University Press, 1981.
4. Lauren Lissner et al. "Dietary fat and the regulation of energy intake in human subjects." *American Journal of Clinical Nutrition,* 46:886–892, 1987.

CHAPTER 10

1. Albert Bandura. "Self-efficacy mechanism in psychological activation and health-promoting behavior," in J. Madden IV, S. Mathysse, and J. Barchas, eds., *Adaptation, Learning and Affect.* New York: Raven Press, forthcoming.

CHAPTER 16

1. Ralph S. Paffenbarger Jr. et al. "Physical activity, all-cause mortality, and longevity of college alumni." *New England Journal of Medicine,* 34:605–613, 1986.
2. American College of Sports Medicine. *Guidelines of Exercise Testing and Prescription.* Philadelphia: Lea and Febiger, 1986.

CHAPTER 17

1. Clive Wood. "Buffer of hardiness: An interview with Suzanne C. Ouellette Kobasa." *Advances,* 4:37–45, 1987.
2. H. Benson. *The Relaxation Response.* New York: William Morrow, 1975.
3. C. Patel. "Randomized controlled trial of yoga and biofeedback in management of hypertension." *Lancet,* 2:1053–1055, 1973.
4. Ilan Kutz et al. "Meditation and psychotherapy: A rationale for the integration of dynamic psychotherapy, the relaxation response, and mindfulness meditation." *American Journal of Psychiatry,* 142:1–8, 1985.

Index

355

Index of Recipes

367

Made in the USA
Coppell, TX
03 December 2020

42814927R00203

"A Friendlier Pritikin... Inviting Lifetime Commitment."
—KIRKUS REVIEWS

THE NEW PRITIKIN™ PROGRAM is at the forefront of medical research, leading the way to a healthier, longer life. This spectacularly successful plan has already helped tens of thousands of people at the Pritikin Longevity Center. It can help you:

- Lose weight without getting hungry or counting calories
- **Lower your cholesterol as much as 25% in 21 days**
- Eat a broad range of delicious foods—with zesty, easy-to-prepare meals and recipes for today's life-styles
- **Dine out healthily**
- Understand the truth about the latest dietary trends—from niacin to olive oil to vitamin supplements
- **Start and stick to a sensible, easy-to-follow exercise program**
- Reduce stress and create a better balance in your life

Designed for a new generation of health-conscious Americans, this state-of-the-art program incorporates the wealth of findings made in the last decade. Whether you have a specific health problem, such as high cholesterol or high blood pressure, or simply want to feel more energetic, will help you live in a healthier way—and feel great every day of your life!

"The recipes...look well-seasoned and appealing...and the whole mood of the book, which includes an ample section on dining out, is one of flexibility." **—CHICAGO SUN-TIMES**

"Not A Diet, A Lifetime Eating Plan."
—WASHINGTON TIMES

$20.95 US / $24.00 CAN

ISBN 978-1-4165-8576-3
ISBN 1-4165-8576-1